CW01513181

Modern Bodybuilding

MODERN
BODYBUILDING

A Complete Guide
to the Promotion of Fitness
Strength and Physique

by

OSCAR HEIDENSTAM

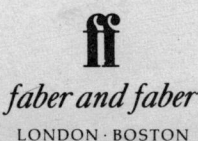

faber and faber

LONDON · BOSTON

First published in 1955
by Faber and Faber Limited
3 Queen Square London WC1N 3AU
Second edition 1957
Third edition 1969
Reprinted 1971, 1978, 1982 and 1985

Printed in Great Britain by
Whitstable Litho Ltd, Whitstable, Kent
ISBN 0 571 06740 9 (Faber paperbacks)

Dedicated to
C.K.E.

Foreword

by John C. Colson, F.C.S.P., M.S.R.G., M.A.O.T.

(*Director of Rehabilitation, Pinderfields General Hospital, Wakefield*)

For many years bodybuilding methods of physical training have been practised enthusiastically by thousands of men of all ages and all nationalities throughout the world. It has not been until comparatively recent years, however, that competent authorities have fully recognized the value of bodybuilding techniques in the fields of physical education, athletics and sport.

Largely this slow recognition has been due to the unscientific 'mumbo-jumbo' background of much of the teaching given in bodybuilding methods, and the dearth of sound reference books on the subject.

This book on modern bodybuilding fulfils a long-felt want; it is authoritative, rational in its outlook, and completely practical and down-to-earth in its teaching. The author is well qualified to write on this subject; he has not only had a very wide experience of all aspects of bodybuilding, but (what is equally important from the reader's point of view) he knows how to impart his knowledge in a clear and concise manner.

Everyone who is interested in muscle training and development will find this book of interest and value. It should certainly be read by all bodybuilders (for whom it will probably become a standard reference book), and by trainers and coaches of athletics and all forms of sport, physical educationists, remedial gymnasts and physiotherapists.

JOHN C. COLSON

Contents

Foreword by John Colson   *page* 9

Introduction—Why Not Join the Fit Set?   15

1. Your Health   17
2. The Age Factor   20
3. Are You the Type You Think You Are?   25
4. What Makes a Muscle Flex?   29
5. Facts to Chew Over About Diet   38
6. What Shape are You Really In?   45
7. How to Exercise Without Equipment—It's Free   54
8. A Gym at Home   69
9. How to Use the Equipment   76
10. Training with Weights at Home   97
11. A Vast Choice of Exercises for You   103
12. Join a Health Studio or a Class   127
13. Weights Give the Sportsman that Extra Lift   135
14. Take a Second Look at Your Breathing   156
15. Coming to Terms with Weight Training   158
16. Weight Training for Boys   163
17. Figure Training for Women   168
18. Now Exercise Your Will Power   175

Index   177

Contents

Illustrations

Shapes of Muscles   *page* 31
Range of Movement   33
Three Orders of Levers   35
Freestanding Exercises—Beginners   58
Freestanding Exercises—Intermediate   60
Freestanding Exercises—Advanced   62
The Home as a Gym   71
Simple expander exercises   78
Some apparatus exercises   85
Iron-Boot exercises   89
Chinning Bar, Roman Chair, Wrist Roller   91
Boards, Leg Press, Calf Machines, etc.   94
Bodybuilding Set   99
Barbell and Dumbell exercises 1, 2, 7, 8, 9, 10, 16, 18, 19, 107
    22, 23, 28, 30, 31, 40, 41
Barbell and Dumbell exercises 4, 5, 6, 14, 25, 26, 27, 32, 51 116
Barbell and Dumbell exercises 11, 13, 32, 33, 36, 37, 38,   120
    49, 51

Introduction

WHY NOT JOIN THE FIT SET?

You have just made an astonishing discovery. You now know that muscles are made for work; so you are reading this book to see how to get the best out of them. And that is the reason why I wrote it—to help someone just like you. You have a specially good reason to build up your body to get fit. It might be to play football; to swim; to fence; or to be a future Mr. Universe title winner. Whatever your reason, *Modern Bodybuilding* is a know-how guide to physical fitness just for you. All the most important exercises are explained clearly. All you have to do is select the ones you need and adapt them to your requirements. And that, through a lifetime of bodybuilding teaching, is simply that. Now it's up to you to go on and get the best out of yourself. It's no use saying that if you had tried a little bit harder you might have made it. Give it all you've got and say proudly: 'I made it.'

CHAPTER ONE

Your Health

The great problem of the present day which faces all of us in our highly civilized and artificial society, is how to be successful in our business and social lives without sacrificing our youth and health. It is unfortunately true that many successful business men (and women too) will go to infinite trouble and expense to perfect the machinery of their businesses and yet completely ignore the fact that the 'machinery' of their individual bodies needs care and attention. And the day of reckoning comes when often in their moments of greatest triumph, and when the highest peak of success has been achieved, collapse occurs. How often do we read that a prominent man has been advised, on doctor's orders, to have a complete rest? Or, worse still, that he has been struck down with a coronary thrombosis?

The problem then is how can we to-day ensure a full measure of both health and wealth. It is simply a matter of common sense; it is a matter of recognizing the equal value of health and wealth and of living a life which takes both fully into account.

No one can be a social success if ill-health is his lot. Success in business will elude you if you can't concentrate, if you are nervous, indecisive; if you are dragging a tired body around, when zeal and energy are called for. However you try, you cannot divorce brain from body.

Remember that although the human body is a highly efficient machine it needs constant care and attention. You don't have to make a fetish of it, but for goodness' sake don't ill-treat it beyond repair.

The six great enemies of good health are these, and probably in this order:

1. Faulty diet

That is: insufficient food, overeating, hasty eating, eating wrong and badly cooked food.

2. Inadequate exercise

A walk to the station, a week-end game, household duties, or manual labour, are not sufficient. A planned system of exercise based on your needs and the time available is an absolute necessity.

3. Poor hygiene

Adequate care must be taken of the skin, teeth, feet and hands.

4. Faulty posture

Many occupations put uneven stresses on the body. Sedentary work restricts proper functioning of the lungs and intestines. Regular bodybuilding exercise is necessary to correct these faults.

5. Wrong mental attitude

Circumstance, work and environment may encourage a negative attitude, developing fears for the future, indecision, uncertainty. Regular bodybuilding exercise is necessary to change these states.

6. Bad habits

Too little relaxation, insufficient sleep, over-indulgence in alcohol and smoking, have no place in the life of those who want to be healthy, wealthy and wise.

Your health is the most important thing in your life.

There is no doubt that money is a very useful thing to have around to buy just about everything. But you can't buy good health, or fitness. You can, though, be poor and work for fitness, and in the daily grind with the weights you will improve your health. Little by little just like an invisible mender you will be doing yourself a power of good. It is very like looking at those old photographs of yourself. You think, was that really me? The change is startling.

That's how it is with bodybuilding. Suddenly you are fit enough to realize just how unfit you were before. It becomes clear in many ways. Nothing is too difficult. You concentrate better. Nerves seem to evaporate. You do not have to drag a tired body round any longer. That's it; you're fit. You may think you look the same, though perhaps you weigh less as the paunch has gone.

You are coping with anything life hurls your way. No magic potion can give you this exhilirating feeling. No coloured pills can give you this lift. All you have to do is work for it.

No one is trying to press-gang you into a spartan régime that develops a world champion weightlifter. You merely want to build your body to reach a personally satisfying standard of physical fitness.

It means you must devote a little time, not necessarily every day, but two or three times a week, to regular exercise. It is the finest investment you can make.

Surely this is a small price to pay for health and vitality.

It is noteworthy to-day that hundreds of the leading personalities in politics, business, medicine, entertainment and also the church are appreciating the value of progressive bodybuilding exercise.

The way *you* can plan your future is indicated quite clearly in this book.

CHAPTER TWO

The Age Factor

It is generally agreed that the urge to improve the physique usually comes to young men between the ages of sixteen and nineteen. This is the time when they become aware of their physical deficiencies and have the wish and incentive to do something to rectify the matter. Some, of course, start earlier, depending on their contact with others or whether they get encouragement at home from their parents and relations.

It is very seldom that a boy at school begins to take a really active interest in his physique, because if he is athletically minded, he will have a variety of games and other athletic pastimes to occupy his leisure time. But to-day in some enlightened and progressive colleges and universities definite schemes are being followed to give students strengthening and bodybuilding work. It is our considered opinion that such work will produce excellent results in the formative years, and will offset much of the wearing-down effects which are produced by a too-heavy programme of competitive athletics which demand high standards of endurance.

Unfortunately, for real progress is always slow, it will be some time before the results of such experiments will be widely known and adopted elsewhere. Meanwhile, numbers of young men leaving school, and others, have to work out their physical development plans on their own initiative.

There is no exact age at which to start bodybuilding. You can be a teenager, middle-aged or elderly. All you have to do is follow the advice in this book regarding the exercises. And one tip I urge you to follow is: tailor the exercises to your particular need. Don't rush in and do a routine that is suitable for a champion swimmer when all you want is to lose an executive's paunch. And that same reasoning goes for younger boys, who would be extremely unwise to attempt a schedule which is planned for an older and physically stronger man. Not only does this sort of mistake put an unnecessary strain on you; it may also bruise your enthusiasm. That could be a more serious injury which may take a long time to heal—and there is an extreme possibility that you may not recover from it at all. That would be as disastrous as not doing any exercise at all.

So the ideal age to start bodybuilding is now.

The urge to get fit may hit you at any stage in your life. You may just want to get fit. Or you may want to develop strength. There's no telling when you want to get fit. But when you do start don't rush it; just take it easy at first. Get your body used to the idea of doing exercises which are completely outside the range of everyday muscular movements. Teenagers will easily absorb the different muscular movements. But if you are older then the musculature will be just that bit less responsive. And if you are about thirty then it would be a good idea to have a medical check before you do any really strenuous exercise. This also applies if you once did a bit when you were younger and have now decided to have another go. Or if you are a little bit anxious about podgy ounces and spare tyres. But whoever you are and whatever your bodybuilding requirements, I wrote this book so that you can get fit with a little application in sessions from as little as fifteen minutes or so a couple of times a week.

To help parents on the right track, a special chapter has been added to this book, setting out what the author declares is a safe form of bodybuilding for boys.

It depends entirely on the individual—his heredity, his environment, his inclination and his ambition. Some schoolboys are 'giants' at fifteen, others are still very much 'boys'. Some thrive on physical activity which is anathema to others.

Is there an ideal age when every boy should start? That is a very different question and the answer is definite, providing that the boy's training is carefully supervised, and that his new hobby does not exclude every other form of physical activity. Body-building must never become a be-all and an end-all, especially in the young.

Bodily growth is greatest in early adolescence and we can therefore put the starting figure at a general one of sixteen, providing the boy is normal in every way.

Care must be taken to point out to the boy any minor postural defects and other slight physical deficiencies, so that he can use the new form of training to the best advantage to overcome these. Far too many young fellows are left to plan their own training and often their only object is to see how big they can get in the quickest possible time, without in the least knowing what they are doing. Like everything else, bodybuilding must be planned and a good foundation laid if success is to be assured.

A great deal has been done in recent years to train club leaders and instructors, but there is still a great deal more to be done. Evening institutes provide very cheap facilities.

Experiments have already been carried out with amazing success in introducing progressive resistance exercises into schools, but naturally this has been very carefully supervised.

The danger of weight-training bodybuilding by the uninitiated lies in the fact that it is only human nature to want to see how *much* one can lift, and not how one can lift a weight *correctly*, and how many repetitions one can do.

Accidents through any form of progressive weight training are very rare, but unfortunately if there is ever an accident caused through nothing more than an individual's carelessness, it is the weight training that comes in for a great deal of unfair criticism, and not the individual's foolishness. A young body-builder may go to the doctor with a strain and is asked how he did it, and you can imagine the reactions when he tells the doctor. He never thinks to explain that with his very little experience, he has attempted to see how much he can lift, and that it is his own carelessness that is to blame. A youth who is learning agility never attempts to do a back somersault the first time he gets instruction; if he did, he would risk breaking his neck, yet no one ever condemns agility! However, in recent years, thanks to the help of such organizations as NABBA, the Central Council of Physical Recreation, and other public bodies, who have arranged proper instruction, such criticism is becoming increasingly rare.

There are still many who imagine that if they are over twenty-one and to all intents and purposes appear to have finished growing, then bodybuilding can do little for them. That this is entirely wrong is illustrated by my own personal story. I was nearing twenty-five when I was first initiated into bodybuilding. It should be remembered that I was already fit and took an active part in many other forms of sport. Also, when I did start, methods were far more haphazard than they are to-day, and my efforts were neither planned nor progressive. Yet in spite of all this, I added nine inches to my chest measurement within the first year, and made steady progress well after the forty mark. I still use weights in my fifties.

There is evidence to show that hundreds of men who have let themselves 'go to seed' in the most frightening way, have benefited enormously in health, strength and appearance when they were past the forty-five mark.

Many business men with limited time find modern body-building an ideal way of getting an all-round exercise programme to cover every muscle group, in the minimum of time. A game of golf usually takes up a whole afternoon and so do games of most other kinds, and all these other sports have drawbacks in that their physical effects are rather onesided. But in half-an-hour's well-planned workout on modern bodybuilding methods, a busy man can cover every muscle group in his body and get a thorough toning up. I know of business executives who train with excellent results but once a week.

If you are a person who has always kept fairly fit, and were fortunate enough to start training at an early age, then you can continue for longer than in any other form of sport, both by adjusting your exercises and by cutting down the time of your workout. For a young trained bodybuilder, a three-hour workout on a complex variety of exercises is quite usual, but when you pass the thirty-five mark, you must cut down the number of exercises, picking out those most suitable to your requirements, and you must shorten the time of your workouts. Also, without any complex changes, you can increase or decrease the repetitions and vary the resistance you handle. It is also essential, as one gets older, to maintain mobility and suppleness by doing full range movements, rather than the various specialized movements better left for the younger generation.

Full range movements, with plenty of abdominal and midsection work should allow one to train for as long as one has the inclination. The ideal plan for a man of, say, forty-five years, is to train three times a week for an hour. I have written a separate book for the older man *Fit at Forty—and After*, in which I cover, in great detail, my keep-fit recommendations for the older man.

As one gets older, the fight against the bulge—the abdominal droop—becomes more difficult, particularly if one is a sedentary worker and fond of the good things of life. If a man can get control over this tendency to bulge between the ages of thirty-five and forty, and provided he leads a normal active life, then it will not bother him much later. There is much wisdom in the adage: 'Prevention is better than cure'.

CHAPTER THREE

Are You the Type You Think You Are?

Take a good look at yourself. Look around you—on a crowded beach, for instance—and you will see men and youths of many different shapes in endless variety. Just as no two sets of finger prints are identical, so are no two bodies exactly alike. You will see thin men, muscular men, fat men. You will see energetic men and lazy men. You will see men with thin upper bodies and thick legs, you will perhaps pity the men with sagging abdomens, fat arms and pipe-stem legs.

You may see young fellows of fifteen and sixteen years old, not less than six feet tall and weighing as much as twelve and a half stones, and boys of the same age less than five feet six inches and hardly turning the scale at nine stones.

Yes, man is moulded in infinite variety to-day just as he was more than two thousand years ago, when Hippocrates studied him and came to the conclusion that although every man was different from the next, he did come within certain categories or 'types'. He believed that a man's temperament was influenced by his physical make-up. He recognized four 'chemical' groups which he called the choleric, the sanguine, the phlegmatic, and the melancholic.

Little more is known of the 'classification of physique' or the experiments in body type and temperament until Dr. William H. Sheldon of Harvard University, a leading exponent of anthropometry, devised a unique plan of measuring the physical structure and relating it to the known temperament. By careful examination of several thousand students at the university, photographing them from front and back and in profile on a standard scaled background, he propounded his theory of Anatomic Type. After a careful consideration of his evidence he went further and claimed that he could identify not more than *three* extreme types. The rounded pear-shaped physique, the pudgy type, he called ENDOMORPH; the muscular athletic he classed as MESOMORPH, and the thin-skinned, fat-less, nervous type got the label ECTOMORPH. The names are in standard use to-day throughout the world.

Let us for a moment look at the recognizable characteristics of each type and try to see in which group you can place yourself, for it is of considerable importance.

The endomorph or 'abdominal' type has usually a characteristic 'roundness' in head and body; has often large bones which are always well rounded with fat. He has a wide short thorax and a long round abdomen. It is said that as his small intestine is 23–35 feet long and his large intestine 5–8½ feet, food has a much longer distance to travel and that more nourishment is derived from it. In disposition he is cheerful and placid, he eats well and often and has difficulty in keeping his bodyweight under control. He is the type which has a tendency to run to fat.

It is obvious that his bodybuilding needs—his training plans —differ from the other types; it is obvious that he must follow a scheme which constantly keeps his interest at a high pitch. It is also obvious that he must train for longer periods than the others.

His extreme opposite, the ectomorph, or 'Thoracic', is usually a touchy, talkative, nervous individual—a bundle of energy. His head is egg-shaped, his features angular. He has thin bones and hardly a scrap of superfluous flesh. His is the long powerful thorax, the capacious lungs and small abdomen—the ideal build for a champion long-distance runner. He likes his meals daintily served and tempting, for his appetite is small. Because he is constantly using up energy, his training must be based on short, intensive periods that require maximum effort over a short period. He must learn to relax. That is his most difficult task, yet when once accomplished, he takes on the happier disposition and potentiality of a 'muscular' type.

The mesomorph, or 'Intermediate', although he may have a leaning towards one or other of the two extremes, is nevertheless a clear-cut type of his own. He is the real manly type, adept at games which require strength more than finesse or skill. He is the solid, reliable type, more staid in character and more normal in habits and dietary requirements. He is the type which responds most quickly to planned exercise. He is what bodybuilding experts call 'the quick gainer'. He makes progress on any form of exercise but does very much better—and more quickly—on a planned system. From his group come, with one or two exceptions, most of the world's leading athletes and sportsmen.

To know to which type you belong is therefore helpful, but it is not the whole story. Environment, daily habits, occupation, all play important parts.

Modern bodybuilding teaches that while no man can completely change his 'type' which was laid down at birth (or earlier) he can tremendously overcome the defects. If he is overweight—or underweight—he can obtain normality. If he is nervous, lacking in self-confidence, he can remedy these conditions surely, safely and easily. In later chapters you will see how it is done.

Because men *are* of different types and temperaments it is thus obvious that their training in bodybuilding will also be different, and why standard, stereotyped courses, while producing good results for some, fail to satisfy others.

Bodybuilding, to be completely successful and satisfying, must be planned individually. A system of training must be tailor-made to suit the individual. It must be a constant experiment to discover which exercises, intelligently planned and intelligently performed, will bring the desired results in the shortest possible time.

Your training for better health and an improved physique should not be looked upon as a penance. It can, and should be, most enjoyable, giving you a feeling of buoyancy and zest. Be enthusiastic about it. Look forward keenly to your next training period and you will not permit yourself to be diverted from the important job you have in hand. And, above all, don't shirk an essential exercise because you can't get the same pleasure from it as you do from others! If it forms part of a definite schedule, prescribed for you in a later chapter, don't neglect it. If you do so you may miss the very exercise which may do you the most good.

The secret of success in bodybuilding lies in the word PRO-GRESSIVE, but there is another word I want you to get to know. It is STICKABILITY.

If you can develop this essential quality of sticking tenaciously to a regular form of exercise I guarantee that you can build a strong and healthy physique.

CHAPTER FOUR

What Makes a Muscle Flex?

It is an astonishing thing that although we live in an Atomic age when nuclear fission, space travel, and supersonic flight are common every-day terms, there is still a very great deal to be learned about the human body. No one can say authoritatively, for instance, how and why muscles *actually* work.

All that scientific experiment has so far discovered is that some kind of impulse, which may be electrical or chemical, produces some kind of action in the minute muscular fibres, causing them to contract and produce movement. And that is not very much more than the physiologist Galvani, of Bologna (1737–98) knew when he saw the twitching of a frog's muscle following the stimulus of an electric current.

There are some experts who support the chemical action theory, for experiment has shown that an 'impulse' to a muscle produces a substance called acetylcholine, which then produces a whole group of chemical changes. Others believe that electrical impulses 'shock' the muscle into action.

Bodybuilders, however, are not greatly concerned about the 'why' of muscle work—they want to know in the simplest possible terms how best a sensible training plan can be compiled to increase their muscular efficiency, their muscular 'tone' and their muscular size.

What Makes a Muscle Flex?

But a knowledge of the fundamentals of muscle work will, however, make their training far more interesting and lead to much valuable personal experiment, and we set out here as concisely as possible the basic features.

First of all, what is muscle? It is the substance of which the body is largely made—almost half the total weight. In addition to the voluntary muscles, i.e. those we activate at the command of the will, the heart, blood vessels and the intestines are also made of muscle. We generally speak of the body as consisting of 'flesh'—and flesh is muscle. The meat we eat consists mainly of the muscle of animals.

Most muscles go in pairs, one on either side of the body. There are 261 (some experts reduce this to 215) of these pairs and five single muscles. Muscles are attached to bone by tendons or aponeuroses (flattened sheet tendons) at both ends. Each muscle has an ORIGIN and an INSERTION. When a muscle contracts—and thus shortens—it will pull the two bones to which it is attached closer together. But usually one bone offers more resistance than the other and so it is the other bone that moves. The muscle is conventionally said to have its origin on the bone that remains still, and its insertion on the bone that generally moves. When it works the other way about (as most muscles do on occasions) it is said to work with origin and insertion reversed.

Muscles move joints solely by virtue of the fact that they pass over joints; and most of them pass over more than one. Often the origin of a muscle is just below another; and the principal action of the muscle is generally on the lower joint.

Before we pass on to the action of muscles, there is still a little more you should know about them: They are of three kinds: VOLUNTARY, INVOLUNTARY (mainly to be found internally) and CARDIAC (pertaining to the heart).

Muscles are made up of hundreds of minute protoplasmic

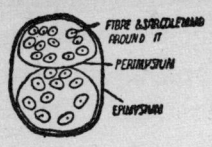

cells arranged in thin fibres. Surrounding each fibre is a protective sheath called the SARCOLEMMA. In turn, bundles of these fibres are covered with a connective tissue called the PERIMYSIUM and groups are further bound together in a tissue called the EPIMYSIUM.

These groups take on various shapes and are sometimes named accordingly. Some are square or rectangular, some round and some have geometrical shapes such as triangles, etc.

A few of the shapes are shown here.

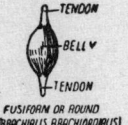 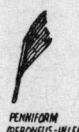 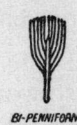 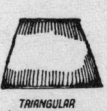 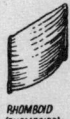

FUSIFORM OR ROUND (BRACHIALIS, BRACHIORADIALIS)   PENNIFORM (PERONEUS-INLEG)   BI-PENNIFORM (RECTUS FEMORIS)   TRIANGULAR (PECTORALIS MAJOR)   RHOMBOID (RHOMBOIDS)

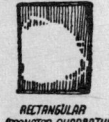 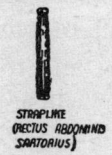

RECTANGULAR (PRONATOR QUADRATUS)   STRAPLIKE (RECTUS ABDOMINIS SARTORIUS)

Muscles are named after their shape, their structure, points of attachment, situation, direction of fibres, action, and size. These are the popular forms.

There are three ways in which a muscle can contract. No muscle is ever quite relaxed and this slight contraction is called muscle 'tone' and involves no movement of the muscle except when some fibres relax and others take over.

When, for instance, you bend your elbow, your BICEPS and BRACHIALIS muscles become steadily shorter and thicker; the muscle moves towards its own centre. This is called CONCENTRIC ACTION. If you lower your arm (i.e. let gravity pull it down) the BICEPS lowers it gradually by slowly relaxing. This is called EC-CENTRIC action. Finally, if you hold your arm with elbow half flexed BICEPS will be contracting but not moving—a static contraction, or since BICEPS stays the same length, an ISOMETRIC contraction. Finally, there are four purposes for which a muscle contracts. It can work as a Prime Mover, Antagonist, Synergist, or Fixator; and as you move about, or perform the simplest movements, dozens of muscles are working all the time in these various capacities.

The muscles that actually perform a movement, as BRACHIALIS and BICEPS in flexing the elbow, are the PRIME MOVERS; and as they contract, their natural ANTAGONISTS (in this case TRICEPS, which extends the elbow) help to keep the movement steady and controlled by gradually relaxing.

But BICEPS also supinates the forearm and flexes the shoulder; and if we wish to flex our elbow without performing these other actions, then the pronators of the forearm and the extensors of the shoulder must also work to inhibit these movements. They work to see that the unwanted tendencies of BICEPS do not prevail—which means that they work as SYNERGISTS.

Finally, if much resistance is offered to the flexing of your elbow (e.g. by a weight) BICEPS will tend to pull down your scapula because it offers less resistance; and to prevent this happening, the upper fibres of TRAPEZIUS will contract to hold the scapula high and fix it—they are acting as FIXATORS.

So many muscles pass over more joints than one that there is always plenty of work for other muscles as synergists; and little less as fixators, for bones are freely movable, and before any muscle can contract at all strongly, it must have its origin securely fixed. In a strenuous exercise for the arms, you tend to hold your breath: your abdominals are holding your thorax still to provide a firm hold for the muscles that originate from it and go to the arms (such as PECTORALIS MAJOR and LATISSIMUS DORSI).

If this sounds very complicated and likely to worry you, work out the exact movement for yourself. If not, dismiss it from your mind; it is not vital to your success.

But what *is* important is that you should know something of how a muscle works *in its range of movement*, and a little about muscle *leverage*.

With your arm at your side, bend your elbow so that your fingers touch your shoulder. The muscles of your front upper arm (BICEPS and BRACHIALIS) have moved from full stretch to full contraction, i.e. through a full range of movement. That is what it is called: FULL RANGE. This is normally divided into two sections known as outer and inner range. In remedial work such a movement is split into three phases, outer, middle and

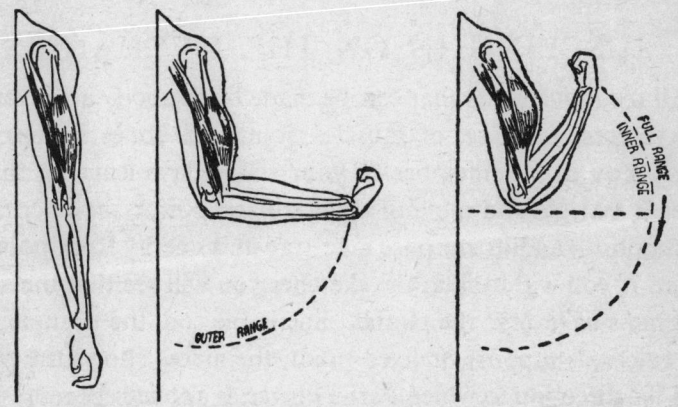

Showing the range of movement of the upper arm

inner Thirds. The accompanying illustration makes this point quite clear.

It is important to know this because modern progressive exercise makes use of these terms in different words, i.e. peak contraction, cramping, etc. (see terms explained).

One of the features of present-day bodybuilding is that much of the muscle-work has been made 'purer', that is to say effort is made to work the muscles individually instead of exercising large muscle groups.

For instance in an upper arm exercise with a weight, it can become a more effective biceps builder if the elbow is rested on a platform or part of the body, thus relieving the shoulders of unnecessary work. Before the advent of squat racks and benches the exerciser (particularly if he practised alone) had to expend a lot of energy in lifting the weights into the starting position for each exercise. It made him stronger, but reduced his capacity for the actual muscle building exercises.

With the use of modern appliances the present-day body-builder can make his training more concentrated, more specialized and more productive of quick results.

MUSCLING IN ON THE MECHANICS

All the movements that can be made by the body are leverage movements. Each set of muscles, joint and bones is simply a lever. You may remember in your schooldays learning that a lever is 'A rigid rod moving about a fixed point', the fulcrum—or support—and its purpose is to transmit energy from point to point. If you will look at the sketches you will see that there are diagrams of levers: the straight line is the rod, the triangle F is the fulcrum, support or fixed point, the arrow shows the place and the direction to which P, the Power, is applied. W represents the weight or the resistance. (Bodybuilders should appreciate that W could be represented as a weight above the rod *or* a cable or spring underneath.)

That part of the lever between Power and Fulcrum is the 'Power Arm'; the part between the Fulcrum and the Resistance is the 'Resistance Arm'. In the diagram they are equal; if the Power Arm is longer than the Resistance Arm, the lever is that much stronger. If shorter, it is weaker and said to work at a mechanical disadvantage. It is unfortunately true that most of our muscles work at a great mechanical disadvantage which prompts the theorists to say that the human body was built for speed rather than strength.

There are three kinds of levers and all are exemplified in the

What Makes a Muscle Flex?

human body with the bones as levers, joints as fulcra and muscles as power.

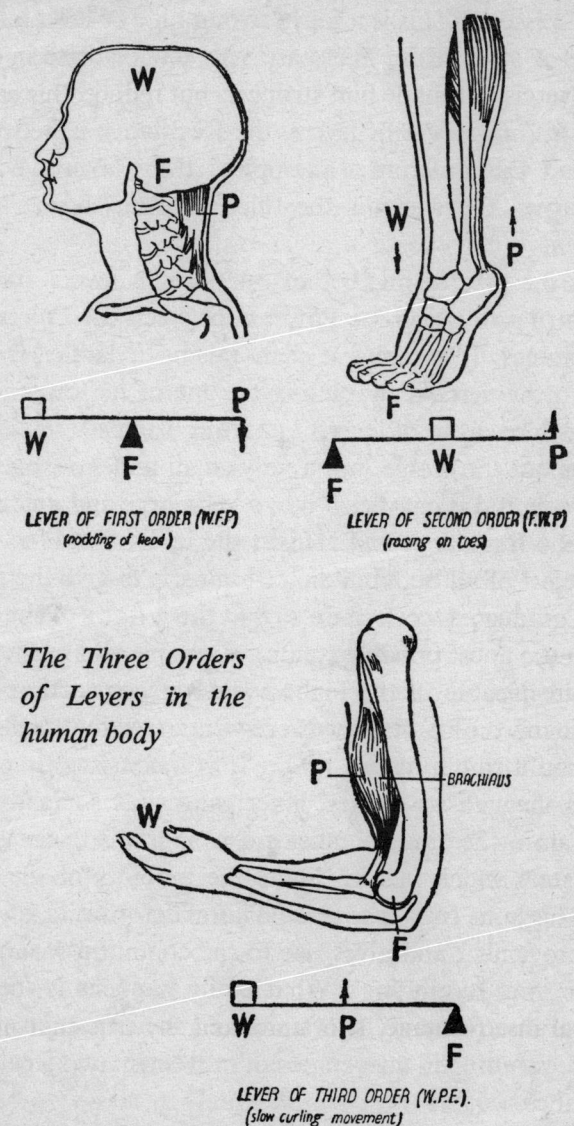

LEVER OF FIRST ORDER (W.F.P.)
(nodding of head)

LEVER OF SECOND ORDER (F.W.P.)
(raising on toes)

The Three Orders of Levers in the human body

BRACHIAUS

LEVER OF THIRD ORDER (W.P.E.).
(slow curling movement)

What Makes a Muscle Flex?

In the *First Order* of levers, the Fulcrum is between the Resistance and the Power. (Examples: see-saw, pair of scales and a pair of scissors.) This is a fairly strong type of lever and earns the name of STABILITY. There are very few of these in the human body.

In the *Second Order* of levers, the Resistance is between the Power and the Fulcrum. (Examples: using a crowbar or a wheelbarrow—the wheel is the fulcrum.) This is the lever of STRENGTH.

By far the greater number of our human levers are of the THIRD ORDER in which the Power is between the Fulcrum and the Resistance. (Example: a man raising a ladder from the ground to the vertical by pulling on one of its lower rungs is using the third order of lever.) Far from being strong, it is very weak and not too stable, but a very small and slow movement at the Power end is converted into a very large and quick movement at the Resistance end. This is the lever of SPEED.

The object of all bodybuilding training is to give the muscles carefully graduated work to do so that the WHOLE of the muscle is kept in the finest possible condition, supple and relaxed when at rest but capable of the highest state of contraction for the work demanded of it. It is therefore vital to see that each muscle is exercised through its full range. If you consistently contract a muscle through its limited inner range—as so many bodybuilders do!—the muscle takes on a shortened, always contracted, state which in turn limits the mobility of the joint it moves. This in its turn produces postural deformities, awkwardness of movement and gives rise to the condition wrongly described as 'muscle-binding'. What really happens is that some muscles are permanently shortened and their antagonists overstretched, resulting in unevenness of movement and weakness in performance.

You can see examples of this shortening and stretching in the poor posture of many workers, particularly those who spend long hours in a cramped position. The office worker bent over a desk which is too low for him develops a rounded back, shortening his chest muscles and stretching the shoulder muscles. As the rounded back upsets the balance of the body a compensatory curve of the abdomen develops giving rise to the condition known as KYPHO-LORDOSIS (rounded back and lumbar forward curve). Then special corrective exercises become necessary.

It is therefore most important that every bodybuilding schedule designed for any purpose should be 'balanced' with stretching and limbering before *and after* intensive muscular contraction work. Typical schedules and training plans are discussed in detail later in this book.

CHAPTER FIVE

Facts to Chew Over About Diet

It seems that everyone is a diet expert; that is why there is so much nonsense written about the subject. No wonder that you become so confused by all you read and often dismiss the subject from your mind because you cannot be bothered to sift the truth. In so doing you may lay up a store of future problems for yourself and certainly prejudice your chances of gaining a fit and healthy body.

An elementary knowledge of diet *is* important to every bodybuilder if he is to make the progress desired, for the simple reason that *diet is important*.

There is a lot of truth in the saying that one man's meat is another's poison. One bodybuilder may thrive on large 'heavy' meals at long intervals, whereas another may do far better on small or 'light meals' at regularly spaced times of the day. Temperament and type come into this matter, for type decides the construction and size of a man's digestive organs, while temperament decides the rate at which the food is consumed and converted or 'metabolized'.

This matter of finding the right sort of food to assist you in your search for physical perfection must therefore be a matter of personal experiment. It is a problem which you must solve for yourself based upon a knowledge of elementary rules of nutrition which we give here in a manner which all can understand.

Food, though in infinite variety, falls into certain groups so far as the dietician is concerned. The main groups are these:

PROTEINS, CARBOHYDRATES, FATS, VITAMINS, MINERALS AND WATER

and we will deal with them in that order.

Protein—a word derived from the Greek *Prôtos*, meaning first—is the most important bodybuilding food. It is the food which not only replaces wear and tear of the muscular tissues (which are themselves stated to consist mostly of protein), but is an energy food as well. It is the only food which contains nitrogen, and as this element is excreted from the body in considerable quantities each day, it must be replaced. Some forms of protein have better bodybuilding qualities than others, i.e. milk, eggs, meat, fish and cheese. These are called 'first class' proteins. In the 'second class' come the vegetable foods, peanuts, the pulses (beans and peas), spinach, carrot and cabbage. A very good source is soya flour (made from the soya bean) which is the common ingredient of some of the much publicized protein foods offered for sale to bodybuilders.

The amount of protein a man requires depends entirely on his body size and the work, including his bodybuilding training, that he does. Scientific study has laid it down that a man in good condition working on a strenuous exercise programme requires about one-thirtieth of an ounce of protein per 2 lb. of bodyweight. It is not easy to work this out: meat, for example—the favourite protein food of bodybuilders—is almost four-fifths water. But we can get some guide. It is stated that one pint of fresh milk supplies about one-quarter of a grown person's daily protein needs. One good portion of meat, fish or poultry adds an equal amount. Two lightly cooked eggs contribute almost a fifth. So with milk, meat, and eggs, as your staple diet, you are still a good bit short of your protein requirement.

It is almost certain that the average bodybuilder in Britain doesn't get enough protein to replace that broken down by strenuous exercise and it is a wise plan to experiment with additional protein foods. Nutritionists advise that it is essential to eat some carbohydrate with protein in the proportion of one carbohydrate to four of protein to get the utmost value. Now that flesh foods are unrationed it is possible to ensure a better intake of protein, and the young bodybuilder is well advised to eat as much as he can afford. All the top-grade athletes of other countries are firm believers in medium-cooked steaks and roasts. Very few top-class athletes relying on strength and stamina for their success are pure vegetarians.

Carbohydrates act as fuel for the engine of the body. In the form of starches or sugars they are stored in the liver, muscles and blood for conversion into energy. Richest sources of starch are the cereals, bread, cereal products, potatoes, and the sugars are in syrups and honeys, ripe fruits, and glucose. Glucose, which by-passes the chemical breakdown in the stomach, is quickly available as energy and it is a wise plan to take a small quantity when it is most acceptable to the body—*after* exercise, when energy reserves are low and when the sugar-content of the blood has been reduced.

Fats are third in our order of essential foods—valuable as heating fuels and reserve energy supply for the body. Available in mineral and vegetable forms, it comes in butter, margarine, oils and cooking fats, fat meat and bacon, milk and cream. It is also found in cheese, nuts, eggs, chocolate and in fish of salmon, sardine and mackerel.

A well-known nutritionist has stated that the above three components of diet should feature in the daily diet of the average bodybuilder in this proportion:

PROTEIN, 4 OZ.; CARBOHYDRATE, 16 OZ.; FATS, 4 OZ.

To keep really healthy, the daily diet requires other things—vitamins, minerals, water and roughage.

Facts to Chew Over About Diet

Vitamins—meaning life-giving substances—are essential to the body. Many have been identified and separated in crystal form. All have their particular purpose, but we need only concern ourselves with those tabulated as A, B complex (a group in themselves), C, D, and E. Briefly:

Vitamin A, essential to health and growth (*lack of it leads to roughening of the skin, night blindness, and lowered resistance to respiratory diseases*), is found in liver, leafy green vegetables, yellow vegetables, i.e. carrots; butter, enriched margarine, cheese, milk, egg-yolk and fruits.

Vitamin B, or the group known as B1 to B12 (*lack of it leads to inflammation of nerves, neuritis, fatigue, indigestion and constipation*) occurs in all the cereals, lean meat, yeast, beans, cheese and some vegetables.

Vitamin C, is commonly called the 'fresh fruit' vitamin, occurring in the citrus fruits, tomatoes, and other vegetables and fruits. (*Lack of it causes rough skins, spongy gums, a tendency to bruise easily, anaemia, and mental depression.*)

Vitamin D has been labelled the 'sunshine' vitamin in that it is created in the body by exposure to the sun. It occurs in eggs, milk and cream, and in irradiated margarine. Fish oils, particularly halibut and cod, are rich in vitamin D. (*Lack of it leads to poor teeth and bones, and serious malformation of the skeleton in young people.*)

Vitamin E is the 'fertility' vitamin, present in wheat germ. Its precise effect on humans is not sufficiently known, because experiment is difficult, but lack of it produces sterility in animals.

While there are many useful vitamin supplements made up in capsule form, it undoubtedly is better for the ordinary person, if he can, to get the essential vitamins from properly prepared food. Not everyone is able, however, to get the right food at the right time, so it may be advisable to supplement the diet with both vitamins and minerals. A careful test will show whether they are worth while.

Facts to Chew Over About Diet

Minerals. Nutritionists have listed thirteen minerals essential to the welfare of the body: calcium, iron, iodine, magnesium, sodium, potassium, phosphorus, sulphur, chlorine, copper, manganese, cobalt and zinc. They are to be found in most foods though it is possible that the two most important, iron and calcium, are lacking in the ordinary diet. As a wise precaution, every bodybuilder should include iron and calcium rich foods. i.e. brown bread and milk in fairly large quantities.

Water and Roughage. About two-thirds of the body's weight is water. It is in every cell and between the cells. It forms the major part of the muscles. Its purpose is to hold chemicals in solution and to permit the vital chemical changes to take place. Insufficient water can cause all sorts of vague pains, lack of appetite, and depression. It is always wise to have a generous intake of fluid every day. In the normal person whose skin and kidneys (both organs of excretion) are functioning correctly, the total fluid intake should *never* be less than three quarts a day. As much of food is water in some form, it means that at least three pints of *liquid* should be taken every day, as milk, water or other beverages. Soda and fizzy drinks, though popular, are not advisable.

Roughage, which is mainly the cellulose of vegetable matter and other fibres, is necessary to correct function of the intestines in that it provides 'bulk' on which the excretory muscles can work. Normal food contains sufficient. In sluggish digestion it may be advisable to increase the bulk by an occasional addition of bran or extra cereals.

That is a brief summary of the essential facts of diet for the bodybuilder. But how is he to apply it to his daily food requirement? These are his *basic* needs daily:

A generous portion of lean meat.

Potatoes and both green and yellow vegetables.

One quart of milk.

One generous serving of cereal.

At least two tablespoonsful of butter or enriched margarine.

A half pint of fruit juice, or juicy fruits.

A helping of fresh uncooked fruit or salad.

Not less than three good slices of brown bread.

Two fresh eggs.

There are two other factors to bear in mind. Meals should be carefully prepared and not ruined by overcooking or reheating. They must be eaten slowly and masticated thoroughly. Whenever possible avoid highly spiced and flavoured 'concocted' meals. Keep away from pastries and synthetic fillings. Try to have your food as natural as possible. No strenuous physical activity should be done less than an hour before, or an hour following, a heavy meal.

By following this advice your body will greatly benefit because the human engine always works better on better fuel.

FOOD SUPPLEMENTS

In spite of higher standards of living in recent years, many people suffer from diet deficiencies through wrong eating, and processed foods.

The chemists' shops and health food stores are doing a vast business in food supplements in many forms. Vitamin pills, halibut oil pills, iron pills, wheat germ, yeast, various types of dessicated liver, protein foods of a thousand varieties. All this to add further confusion to the complex pattern of eating habits.

Like artificial sunlight, food supplements are just that; they are an alternative to a good diet with its full complement of all the necessary vitamins, minerals, etc. to keep you well and fit. But they play a very important and essential part in maintaining good health.

Athletes and people who indulge in regular exercise do need some form of supplements to give them extra protein and to compensate for the extra physical work they do. I recommend good supplements to all who take regular exercise. In the winte months when fresh vegetables, fruit salads etc., all so rich in essential vitamins, are harder to get or more expensive, food supplements are a great asset.

I believe that wheat germ in some form is excellent, particularly for the older man, and athletes should certainly have both wheat germ and some form of extra protein supplement· Do remember, though, that however eye-catching the advertising media may be the system can only absorb a certain amount of protein and other vital vitamins and over-indulgence only means they are eliminated as waste. I once met a woman channel-swimmer who told me that she was taking ninety wheat germ capsules a day! Some top-line bodybuilders indulge in too many types of supplements, far more than their systems can absorb even with the heaviest training schedules. There are also some very poor imitations on the market so always buy reputable brands. Extra protein is not fattening.

Health foods are a vast subject and big business, and there are many magazines and books on the subject alone. So many people ask me what I think of supplements. I think they are essential for the athlete and the person who cannot always eat the correct foods.

CHAPTER SIX

What Shape are You Really In?

THEY'VE GOT YOU TAPED ALL WRONG

Those public weighing-machines on a railway station, or in a chemist's shop, usually show a table of measurements telling you what you should weigh at a certain age and at a certain height. Having paid your money, have you noticed that rarely does your recorded weight coincide with the tables? Let me say at once that the tables are often quite useless. They take no account of the steadily increasing height and weight of the *average* man in the British Isles. They ignore completely a person's body type, and often, through ill-treatment by individuals who will treat them as playthings, give inaccurate figures! These tables were compiled from 'insurance' statistics some time ago and represent an average of a small number of selected persons whose vital statistics of age, weight and height were known.

Weight, height and age are, of course, merely the basic measurements and have really no definite connection with each other. A man does not inevitably get heavier as he gets older, though he may do so as a result of over-eating and under-exercising. You cannot definitely say that one man is underweight because he is tall or that he is overweight because he is short. It is really a matter of body type.

But it is possible to define, according to accepted standards of good physique, the limits of each *kind* of physique taking into account the man's experience of modern bodybuilding training.

I have had long experience in seeing and measuring most of the best-developed athletes in the world, and believe it is feasible and helpful to set down certain standards of physical proportion. These are 'ideal' measurements which a bodybuilder can achieve after, say, six months of progressive bodybuilding.

	Light Build	*Medium Build*	*Heavy Build*
Height	5 ft. 8 in.	5 ft. 8 in.	5 ft. 8 in.
Weight	11 st. 0 lb.	11 st. 7 lb.	12 st. 6 lb.
Chest (expanded)	43 in.	45 in.	47 in.
Waist	29 in.	30 in.	31 in.
Upper arm	14 in.	15 in.	16 in.
Neck	14½ in.	15½ in.	16½ in.
Thigh	23 in.	24 in.	25 in.
Calf	14 in.	15½ in.	16 in.
Wrist	6½—6¾ in.	7 in.	7½—7¾ in.

From this simple table it will be seen that in the three types the ratio of neck–arm–calf is almost identical and this is one of the elementary facts in good proportion. But how many men can say that at a height of 5 ft. 8 in. and a neck measurement of 14½ inches they have a well-developed arm stretching the tape to 14 inches? And how many heavy-built men have a difference between the measurements of expanded chest and waist of 16 inches?

Remember the figures given in this table are not the measurements of the average *man* in Britain, nor of the average bodybuilder. They are ideal measurements which can be achieved by planned exercise. Let us, for a moment, consider the average man, and some well-known facts.

Most made-to-measure suits are cut to a standard pattern and show a difference in chest and waist of less than 4 inches. Many off-the-peg suits allow for waists larger than chests!

What Shape are You Really In?

Judging by the correspondence the author receives there are many hundreds of young fellows anxious to join the police force and who fail because they cannot measure up to the minimum physical standards required. There are thousands of young fellows in the 5 ft. 10 in. height region, who weigh under 10 stone and whose chests measure less than 36 inches. If they are healthy, as most are, a few months on planned exercise will soon alter that!

The average man, too, usually has large hips. In a well-built individual of 5 ft. 8 in. tall, the hips should not be more than 36 to 38 inches. If he is a big man of 6 ft., his maximum hip measurement should not be more than 40 inches.

How can a man tell to which type of body build he belongs? You have had some guidance in the chapter on 'Are you the type you think you are?' But the tape measure can help too.

Potentiality for physical development can be roughly assessed by your bone formation. It is commonly accepted that if you have large and strong bones your capacity for further development is very good. If you have a slim frame with small bones (and plenty of energy too!) your chances of very heavy muscular development are not so great.

How can you tell your bone size? This is usually left to the specialist, but nature can give you help in finding out. Put a tape measure round your wrist where there is the smallest amount of covering of tissue, and where your measurement is closest to the two bones of your forearm. You will record anything from 6 to 8 inches. If your wrist measures less than 7 inches and you have already reached maturity, it is not likely that however hard you train you will ever obtain a massive physique. There are exceptions of course and a few men have developed an outstanding physique in spite of their small bone structure. If, on the other hand, your wrist is large and in the $7\frac{1}{2}$ to 8 inch category, your task in building a fine physique will be much easier.

CHEST MEASUREMENTS

Chests can be measured in various ways and varying results obtained. This fact makes the edict that a man must have a certain size chest before he can enter a public service rather silly. You can have, in a trained athlete, a *deflated* chest of 32 inches which expands to 37 inches or more, thus showing a high state of lung capacity. But it is still, according to modern bodybuilding standards, a *small* chest. You can have also a *normal* chest (neither expanded nor deflated) of 41 inches which when inflated only stretches the tape to 43 inches. This is quite a big chest but the lung capacity is not what it should be.

The ideal to work for is a mobile chest of good size which when deflated is about 38 inches, but when fully expanded, bringing the large muscles of the back (the latissimus dorsi) into contraction, will record something like a total 'expansion' of *10 inches*.

Progressive resistance exercise greatly increases not only the mobility of the whole thorax but by putting additional work on the lungs, greatly increases their efficiency, resulting in increased size of the chest internally and externally.

As every bodybuilder finds it encouraging to progress, to record his gains in measurements as well as appreciating the increased feeling of well-being, it is important that he should take his measurements carefully.

It is not easy to do this ACCURATELY by oneself, although if you cannot get someone to help you, these instructions will enable you to get somewhere near to accuracy.

First of all, draw up a chart as shown on page 53. Record your *age* in years and months. To measure your *height* stand in your bare feet against the wall or edge of a door. Place a ruler flat on your head and as horizontal as you can. Pressing the ruler against the wall or door edge, turn round and mark the

48

position. Measure accurately to floor level. While standing against the wall, try to get heels, buttocks, shoulders and head to touch. (If you can't, your posture is faulty!)

Your *weight* should be taken carefully. If you have no scales get yourself weighed at a chemist's, and immediately you get home, take your clothes off and weigh them on the kitchen scales. Deduct this from the figure given by the chemist and you have your real bodyweight. If you have no kitchen scales, make sure you wear the same clothes when next you are weighed on the same scales at the same chemist's; otherwise your records will be faulty!

If you are flabby and out of condition when you start body-building, you can expect a reduction in bodyweight immediately.

Measure your *neck* at its thinnest part, usually just under the chin and not over your prominent 'Adam's apple'.

Measuring the *chest* is not easy, for it is important to ensure that the tape measure is horizontal all the way round and is not twisted. There should be three measurements— chest contracted (made as small as you can by completely exhaling), chest inflated (simply by inhaling all the air you can), and chest expanded (by which you lift your thorax, widen your shoulders and bring the back muscles to a full state of expansion). The measurement should be taken with the tape across the nipples at the front and level elsewhere.

The *waist* measurement is taken at the level of the navel, when standing normally upright with the chest normally lifted. Don't cheat on this and deliberately make the abdomen as small as possible by drawing it in.

Measure the *hips* across the centre of the buttocks when contracted. It is no true measurement if the buttocks are relaxed as the difference might be as much as 2 to 3 inches.

Two measurements should always be recorded for the upper arm—i.e. Straight and Flexed. The first is taken round the thickest part while the arm is outstretched at shoulder level, muscles relaxed. Flexed measurement is taken with the arm at shoulder level and bent at the elbow with biceps fully contracted.

The *forearm* size is taken with the arm outstretched, fist clenched, at the thickest part.

The *calf* measurement is taken at its thickest part with the muscles contracted, usually by pointing the toes or by lifting one foot off the ground and then pointing the toes, thus contracting the calf muscles.

Ankle and *wrist* measurements are taken just above the protecting bones and not around them.

All the measurements should be taken before you start exercising. By doing so you get what in bodybuilding language are called 'cold' measurements. If you take them during or immediately after a trainnig session, when the muscles are engorged with blood, considerable variations will occur.

Note this important fact too. Gains in measurements are not always regular and progressive. Rapid gains will be made at the start of your training and then may come a period when they stop. You often reach a 'sticking point' at this stage and staleness may intervene. If so, stop training for a week and then return with a new zest.

Quickest gains will come to the chest and arms with increase in bodyweight. It is quite normal to put up to 2 inches on your expanded chest within the first fortnight—but it won't continue at this rate. The author recently had a small wager with a doctor that he could increase his chest measurement by 1 inch during ONE session of weight-training exercise. He was measured before and after by another doctor and in fact increased his expanded chest measurement by *over* 1 inch! Most of the gain was made by the increased mobility of the chest, but he was convinced, and now regularly does his 'stint' twice a week.

SOME FACTS ABOUT 'STAR' BODYBUILDERS

Although, of course, he had a terrific initial potential, Arnold Schwarzenegger of Austria won amateur and professional universe titles by the time he was 21. He had, at that age and at 6 ft. 2 in., a 58-inch expanded chest, a 21-inch flexed upper arm, and weighed 250 lb. But even he had trained for six years to achieve this.

Reg Park, Britain's greatest ever bodybuilder, built himself an upper arm in two years that was bigger than his thigh measurement when he started. At forty he was in as good a physical shape as he was at twenty-two.

Steve Reeves, a former Mr. America, won a Universe title in 1950 and then went on to make a fortune in the Hercules-type films which were popular for a time. Twenty years later he is still considered the ideal of many body-conscious enthusiasts.

John Citrone of Co. Durham, at 5 ft. 5 in. and weighing 168 lb, did a Bench Press (a routine bodybuilding exercise) with nearly 500 lb. John is now a professional strongman and his act is reminiscent of the old time strongmen in their heyday.

Popular feat of top bodybuilders is to inflate and burst a new hot water-bottle. This calls for terrific lung power and stamina, as the feat can take over ten minutes to accomplish if the bottle is a really good one.

People who imagine that top musclemen are not strong are very wrong; they have tremendous strength in all the types of lifting exercises they carry out in their training. Many top musclemen turn to professional wrestling, and of course many of our top lifters have also concentrated on bodybuilding.

The author, although heading for sixty, still trains three times a week and is actually handling weights as heavy as he did at any time in a long career.

What Shape are You Really In?

Do remember that the top musclemen are 'specialists' and you should never take a specialist in any sport as a typical example of that sport.

This is a highly specialized age, and to reach the top in any form of athletic endeavour, you cannot afford to be versatile in several sports whatever your choice may be.

Date	Measures	Date	Increase	Date	Increase	Total Increase
AGE						
WEIGHT						
HEIGHT						
NECK						
CHEST						
Contracted:						
Normal:						
Expanded:						
WAIST						
HIPS						
UPPER ARM						
Straight:						
Flexed:						
FOREARM						
WRIST						
THIGH						
CALF						
ANKLE						

If you are interested in recording the details of your progress, a chart similar to the above is useful.

CHAPTER SEVEN

How to Exercise Without Equipment—It's Free

You may believe that because you have an active job, play games regularly, and get other recreation at week-ends, you are doing enough 'exercise' to keep yourself fit. This is a common and erroneous belief. First of all it is very difficult to assess the *standard* of fitness you achieve and, secondly, most games and sports break down the body rather than build it up and in many cases are but activity for one side of the body only, resulting in uneven development and the creation of stresses and bad posture.

Every player should ensure that additional exercise is taken to preserve the balance of the body. This is best done by the regular practice of one of several forms of exercise.

For the man or woman who wants to achieve a high state of health and fitness, for the week-end sportsman who wants to be on top of his game, for the athlete who requires some building up and work not possible during his athletic training, there is nothing better than a planned system of training.

You can do freestanding exercises in the bedroom or in the garden, in the club or the gymnasium. Get out of your mind the idea that they are PHYSICAL JERKS. The term is as out-of-date as 'horse-buses'.

Modern callisthenics, or freestanding exercise, is a system of smooth, rhythmical movements designed to give the body suppleness, speed, stamina and co-ordination. Because of this fact, this form of training does not aim to, nor does it produce great increases in strength and size in the muscles. Its main aim is to keep the body in a good state of health and muscular tone. But it does form ideal preparatory work for anyone whose ambition it is to build a more-than-average physique with an higher-than-average degree of strength.

In applying the exercise schedules which follow, it is important to see that they are correctly followed if the maximum benefit is to be obtained.

A good exercise plan is usually divided up something like this:

1. An active exercise such as running on the spot, astride jumping, skip jumps, etc., to get the circulation generally speeded up.

2. An arm and shoulder exercise for mobility.

3. Trunk exercises including dorsal and lateral exercises for trunk and dorsal strength and mobility.

4. Abdominal exercises. These are most important for everyone.

5. Leg work for co-ordination and balance and stamina.

6. A breathing exercise, to normalize breathing and circulation.

How many exercises of each type you have in one session depends on the time at your disposal.

For remedial purposes this form of non-apparatus exercise is widely used, particularly for postural defects, foot exercises, and post-operational conditions. I am including separately in this chapter a few general exercises for posture correction whether the defect is lordosis or hollow back, kyphosis or round back, or scoliosis or lateral curvature, or a combination of both. The exercises I have given are general posture correction exercises.

I have also included a short schedule of foot corrective exercises which I hope will be beneficial to those who suffer from tired feet and minor defects.

The great disadvantage of freestanding exercises is that progression in strength, stamina and actual bodily development are limited.

There are of course countless exercises, but the range of progress is limited. The only way to progress, i.e. increase the severity of the exercise so that the body is encouraged to respond, is by increasing the number of times the same exercise is done, but this would lead to fatigue and monotony, which is not a good thing. Progression *is* possible, but only in about four stages. For example in an exercise like Prone Lying Chest Lift off Floor, progression is made by altering the position of the arms, i.e. hands on hips, neck rest and arms above head. These are three forms of progression, but after that what can be done? A new exercise must be found that is harder.

I am giving you three simple freestanding schedules which are well balanced and progressive. The schedules should be combined later with those we recommend for resistance work, particularly the abdominal group. You can also select some of these exercises as a warm-up for the weight-training schedules, and also for the athletic and sports exercises.

A few separate exercises especially for the mid-section are also detailed as so many people are concerned principally with this area.

It is important for the reader not to confuse these schedules, which are for the individual, with any type of Physical Training lesson given in class formation. The latter is quite a different matter and outside the scope of this book.

Here then are your tables:

SIMPLE EXERCISES
WITHOUT EQUIPMENT

TONING UP—BEGINNER

1. Feet together, arms at side—Rhythmic arms swing forward and upward with heels raising on upward swing, lowering on downward. Repeat 20 times.

2. Standing—Alternate knee raise high to chest and grasp with hands, pulling knee to chest. Keep free leg straight and body upright. Repeat 12 times each leg.

3. Standing feet astride—Relaxed trunk bending downward to touch floor with hands in front of feet and between legs as far as possible. Upward stretch and repeat, keeping legs straight, and heels flat on floor. Repeat 12—15 complete movements.

4. Feet astride hands on hips—Trunk relaxed bending from side to side. Ensure body is kept upright and elbows and shoulders well back. Repeat 12 times each way.

5. Front support (on the hands down). Arms bend and stretch. Keep body in a straight line, and avoid sag in the middle. Repeat two sets of 8—12 repetitions, according to capabilities.

6. Prone lying (face downwards) hands on hips—From position of exercise above lower to this position. Chest and head lift high off floor. Inhale on lift, exhale on lower. Feel shoulder blades meet on lift. Repeat 12—15 times.

7. Back lying, palms of hands flat on floor at sides—Knees raise high to chest and lower under control. Repeat two sets of 8 repetitions or more, with rest in between each set. Don't hold the breath!

8. Front support (on the hands down)—Alternate foot place forward and back, getting knee well between arms. Keep arms straight and no body sag. Repeat 12 times each leg.

9. Light skipping on toes with high knee raise. No rope necessary. About 30 seconds.

10. Standing, hands on hips—Quick full knees bend and stretch, keeping heels flat on floor. Hold on chair if balance is difficult. Repeat up to 15—30 repetitions.

11. Back lying, knees raise, feet flat on floor and hands at sides. Relax completely and draw abdomen in, breathing out deeply and in deeply through the nose. Try to feel whole of spine—particularly lumbar area—against floor. Draw abdomen in as much as possible as you breathe out, keeping back flat on the floor.

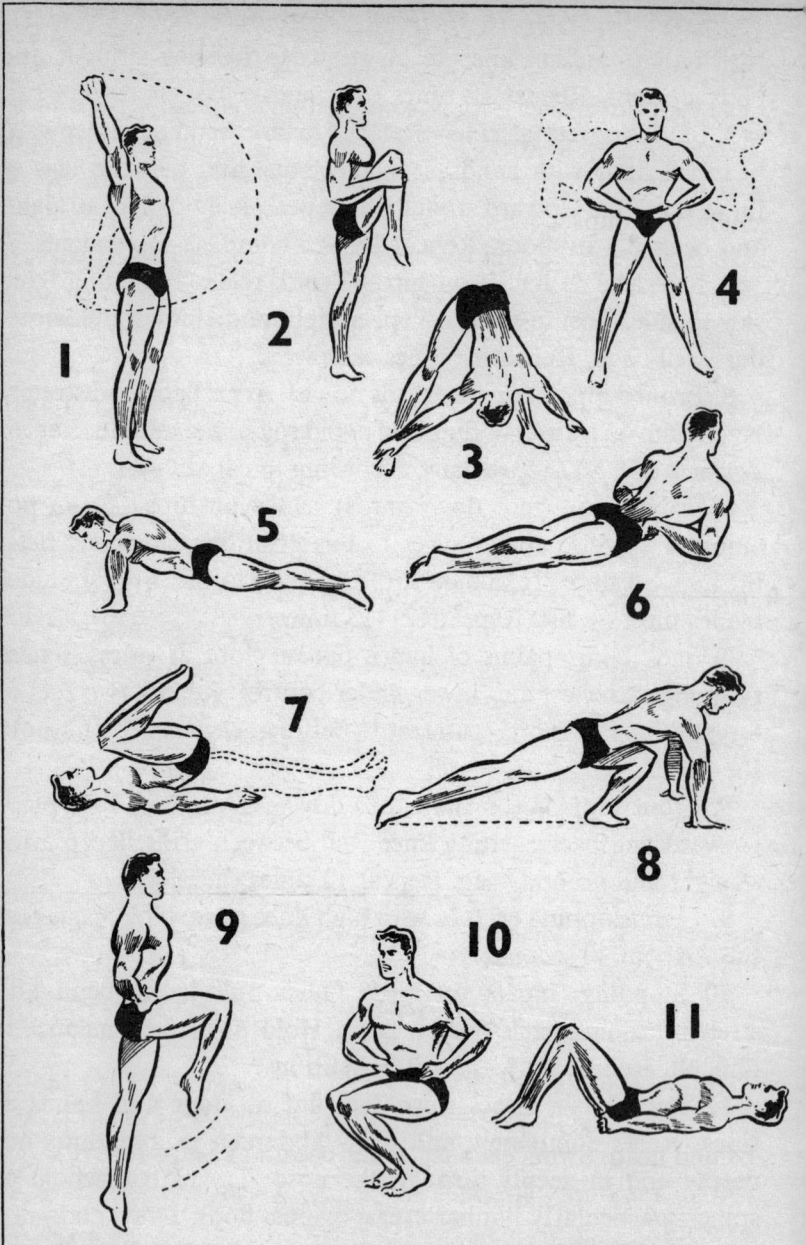

FREESTANDING EXERCISES—BEGINNER

TONING UP—INTERMEDIATE

1. Astride—Arms swinging upward with shoulder press back. Every third upward swing, jump upwards forcing the feet back but not bending the knees. Thirty complete movements to include 10 jumps.

2. Stand astride, trunk relaxed—forward bend and grasp opposite ankle with both hands, and pull head towards knee. Legs must be kept straight. Twelve times each side.

3. Stand astride, arms at neck rest—trunk bending from side to side freely with head relaxed. Keep chest well up and arms well back, shoulder blades together. Ensure that there is no forward movement of the body. Repeat 12 times each side.

4. Front support (on the hands down), jump to crouch and back. Keep knees together and inside arms. Repeat 12 times and increase as progression is made.

5. Prone lying—grasp ankles and lift head, chest and trunk as high as possible. Relax and repeat several times. Breathe in as lift is made, out as you relax.

6. Front support with feet on chair or box, hands on floor (on hands down). Arms bend and stretch, without sagging the body. Repeat two sets of up to 15 repetitions each set.

7. Back lying, arms above the head—legs raise straight, and try to touch floor behind head, without bending knees. At first merely raise legs as far as possible. Repeat two sets of 8—12 repetitions.

8. Back lying, arms above head—trunk raise to forward reach, trying to put head on knees without bending them. Repeat 12—15 times and increase to two sets. Fix feet under heavy object.

9. Back lying, hands on hips—alternate leg swing to touch floor behind head. Swing each leg as far back and as far forward as it will go each time, keeping legs straight. Carry on for about 30 seconds.

10. Skip jumps with high knees raise on every third jump Repeat 15 complete times.

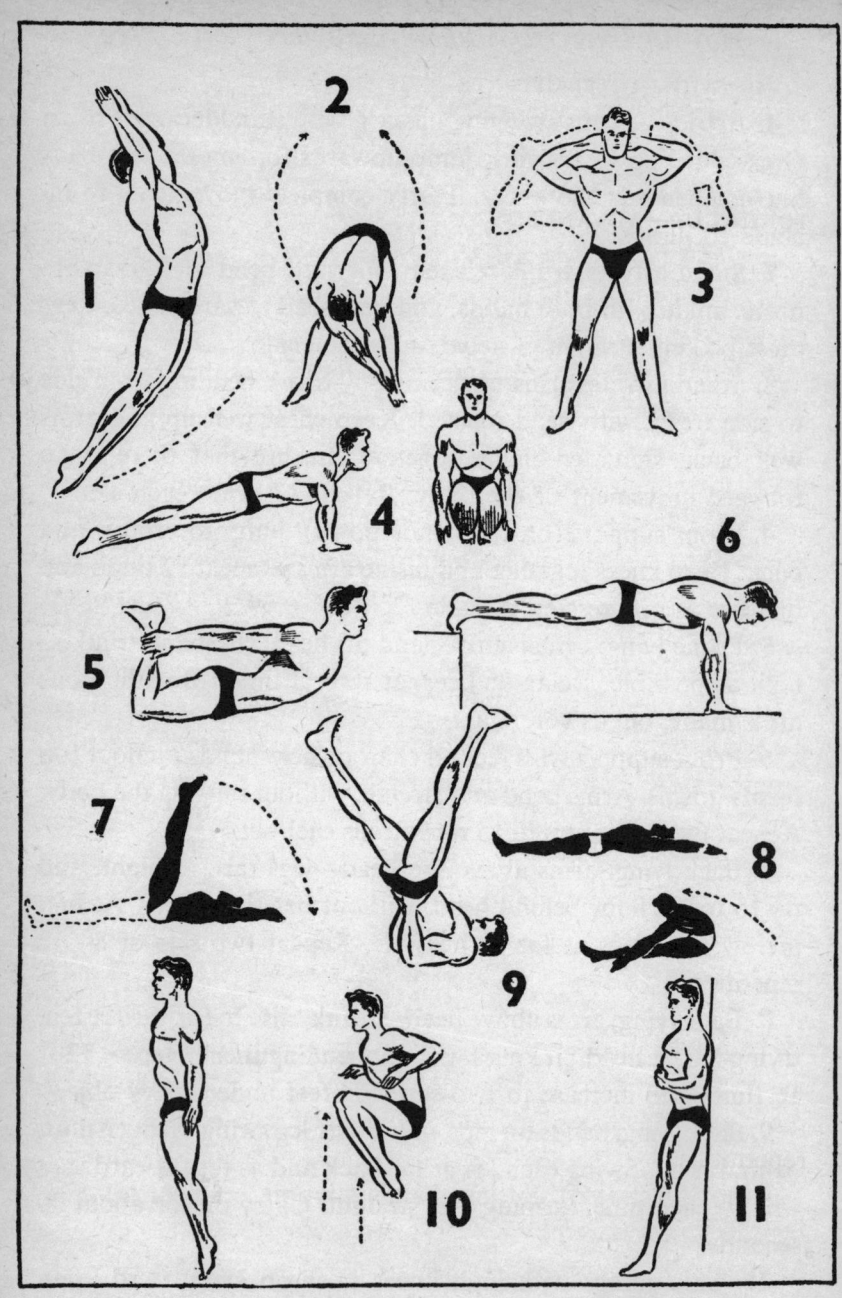

FREESTANDING EXERCISES—INTERMEDIATE

11. Stand relaxed against wall, feet about 24 inches forward and together—practise chest lifting (keeping the abdomen tucked in) with deep breathing.

TONING UP—ADVANCED

1. Stand feet astride, arms to sides—Arms swing forward, extend sideways with shoulder press and lower. Repeat rhythmically 20 complete times.

2. Stand feet together, knees straight—quick relaxed trunk bending downwards to touch floor with hands, and upward stretch. Try and put palms of hands on floor, and let head move freely to try and touch head on knees. Repeat 20 times.

3. Stand astride, arms above head, fingers interlocked, shoulders well back—Trunk bending from side to side freely, keeping hips square to front, arms locked, and body completely straight. Repeat to count of 30.

4. Prone lying, neck rest. Chest, head and legs lift off floor to form bow shape with body. Ensure legs are kept straight and arch comes from head, chest and back. Lower and repeat. Inhale on lift, exhale on lower. Repeat 15 times.

5. Back lying, arms sideways, palms of hands flat on floor. Alternate leg raise to right angles with body, carry over to touch opposite hand with foot. Return leg to upright and lower. Repeat alternate legs. Shoulders must be kept flat on floor, and hips not carried over too far. Repeat 12 times each leg.

6. Back lying, arms above head. Trunk and legs raise simultaneously to form V position with body, and touch toes with hands. Lie back and repeat. Balance may be difficult at first, and movement must be done quickly. Repeat two sets of 10—15 repetitions.

7 (not illustrated). Sitting, hands support on floor, elbows locked. Knees raise high to chest and lower slowly. Try to keep body upright and do not lean back *too* much. Repeat two sets of 10—15 repetitions.

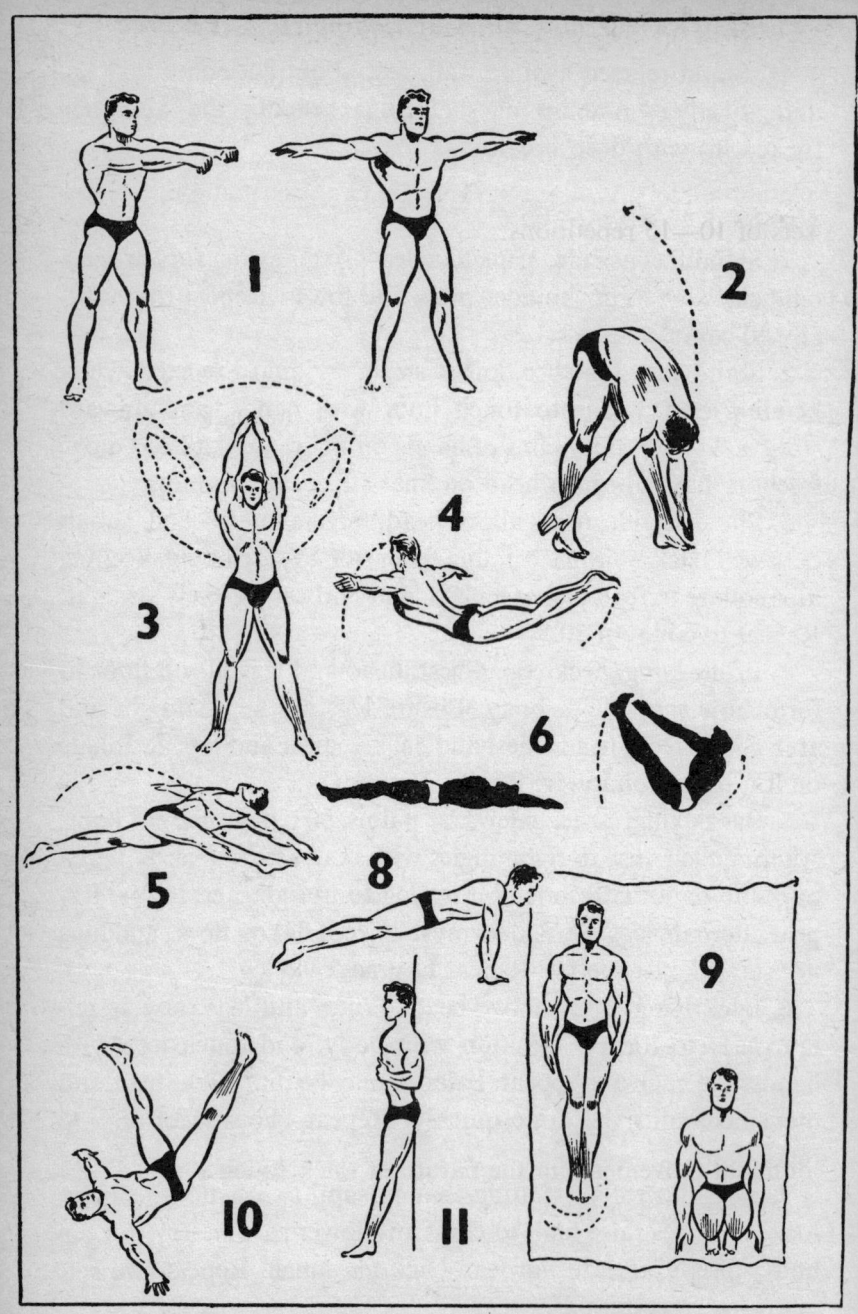

FREESTANDING EXERCISES—ADVANCED

8. Front support (on the hands down) done with feet and hands on chairs or boxes to form a triangular base. Chairs fairly wide apart. Arms bend and stretch getting as low as possible with shoulders, without sagging body in the middle. Try two sets of 10—15 repetitions.

9. Skip jumps to crouch position, knees together every third jump.

10. Back lying, arms above head. Legs raise 45 degrees, legs parting as wide as possible and closing. Repeat 15 times.

11. Lean against wall, feet forward 24 inches and together. Deep breathing. Try and feel whole of spine against wall. Draw abdomen in as far as possible on completion of exhalation. Repeat several times.

SIMPLE EXERCISES FOR THE WAIST-LINE

Although I have included three complete freestanding schedules which can be followed by most young people, there are many older folk who are more interested in an exercise plan to reduce accumulated fat round the mid section. So I will include a few extra exercises specially arranged to deal with this adipose tissue.

Do remember that for sluggish mid sections it is not only necessary to do some form of 'abdominal' exercises but also lateral, twisting and circular movements, as quite as much surplus fat accumulates at the sides and back of the waist line as round 'the bulge' itself.

In the freestanding schedules I have given quite a few abdominal movements in the nature of Back Lying Knees Raise, Legs Raise, Legs Swinging with hips support, also sidebends of many types, but do remember that exercises in the nature of front support and prone lying (where the whole abdomen is lifted) have a marked effect.

When one is in the front support (on the hands down position) the abdominal muscles are contracted to support the body. Here are a few exercises not included in the freestanding schedules:

1. Back lying, hips support—Cycling action with legs. Try this in vigorous and slow bursts.

2. Back lying, arms above head, with feet held on low box about 12 to 18 inches high. Trunk raise to forward reach.

3. Back lying, legs raise to touch floor behind head, support hips with hands, then try and move feet left and right two or three steps in each direction whilst in this position. This is a very advanced exercise not suitable for those who have not toned up their mid section.

4. Back lying, hips support. Legs parting and closing as wide as possible.

5. Cat stretch. In the front support, i.e. hands down position, lean forward, raise hips high and lean back—following the movements of a cat stretching.

6. Stand astride, hands on hips, trunk twist left and right trying to keep hips square to front.

7. If you can find a broomstick or bar try this. Standing, feet astride, arms stretched sideways along stick. Trunk twist from left to right. Also in this position try trunk bending from side to side, keeping body upright.

8. Stand astride, arms above head, fingers interlaced. Trunk circling completely to first left and then to right.

9. Hanging on a bar or beam, knees raise to chest. Also later legs raise. Both are excellent exercises.

10. Stand astride, one foot on a chair sideways on. Trunk bend side to side. Progression to neck rest, also arms above head.

POSTURE EXERCISES

To be taken very gradually two or three times a week, with plenty of breathing space between exercises.

How to Exercise Without Equipment—It's Free

1. Standing, arms forward, fingers stretched—Arms swing sideways with shoulder press, maintaining position of body with no forward or backward movement. Repeat 15 times.

2. Stand astride, arms upward swing in three movements, forward, midway and upward, and shoulder press on third count. Ensure body remains rigid and no backward movement. Repeat 15 times.

3. Stand astride, arms at sides. Relaxed trunk bend down to touch palms of hands on floor, or as near as possible, ensuring that there is no knee bend. Trunk unroll slowly to upright position. Repeat 12 times.

4. Stand astride, arms across bend, fingers straight. Alternate arm swing sideways with trunk and head twist. Endeavour to keep hips square to front. Repeat to count of 20.

5. Stand feet together. Alternate knee raise high to chest grasping knee with hands. Keep rear leg straight, and pull knee as high as possible to chest. Repeat 8 times each side.

6. Back lying, arms above head. Alternate knee raise high to chest. Repeat 8 times each side.

7. Back lying, arms out sideways, palms of hands flat on floor. Chest and head lift off floor by pressing palms of hands on floor Inhale on lift, exhale on lower. Repeat 12 times.

8. Prone lying, hands on hips. Chest and head lift off floor. forcing shoulders well back. Inhale on lift, exhale on lower.

9. Standing with hand on chair for support. Alternate leg swing forward and back as far as possible, keeping leg straight and toe pointed. Repeat up to 10 times each leg.

10. Stand astride, neck rest. Trunk bend from side to side freely, keeping shoulders well back and body upright.

11. Back lying, palms of hands on floor, knees raised and feet flat on floor. Relax completely and breathe out, feeling the whole of the spine against the floor. Inhale deeply through nose, and exhale completely through nose, drawing abdomen well in.

TONE UP THE FEET MUSCLES

If your feet are really flat and have been diagnosed as such by your doctor, there is little you can do. If there is no muscular pain in your feet, then they are better left alone.

However, if you are standing all day, or carrying a lot of surplus weight, the muscles in your feet will need toning up. Without going into a great deal of technical detail on the mechanics of the feet, here are a few simple exercises you can use to keep your feet in good condition. Exercises to be done with bare feet, and if possible, of course, in warm surroundings.

1. Sitting on chair—alternate foot raise off floor and ankle rotate outwards pointing toes. Complete five or six complete rotations outwards, and then the same inwards, with each foot. Do this several times over. A slight cramp may be felt at first; if so, rub the feet.

2. Sitting, feet flat on floor, toes pointing to front—with heels on floor and pads of toes on floor, foot arching by pressing toes and heels on floor. Repeat about 15 times.

3. Support on wall or piece of furniture and standing, feet short astride, toes to front—heels raise off floor as high as possible and lower. Repeat 20 times.

4. Standing, feet short astride, with some support for balance —rocking forward on to toes and back on to heels, lifting toes off floor when rocking back. Repeat 20 times.

5. Walking on the heels, toes pointing to front—across room and back two or three times.

6. Sitting, feet short astride, toes to front—rub sole of one foot on instep of other in circular movement left to right. Repeat several times each foot.

7. Sitting, feet flat on floor, toes to front—lift toes only off floor and try to spread them, then lower and try to pick small object off floor with foot. Repeat several times.

8. Sitting one leg across knee, grasp heel with one hand and upper part of foot with other. Twist upper part of foot upwards to see sole, holding the heel stationary. Repeat several times each foot.

9. Sitting—ankle shaking with foot completely relaxed.

Hygiene of the feet is necessary. They should be washed in warm water daily, and plunged into cold after. Dry carefully and dust with talcum powder. A tendency to Tinia (foot fungus) needs careful attention as it is very contagious. Give your feet air by removing shoes and socks as often as possible, especially in hot weather.

RESISTANCE EXERCISES WITHOUT APPARATUS

When we talk about 'Resistance' exercises it is usually understood that some appliance or special equipment provides the resistance against which the muscles work. But there are some forms of self-resistance exercises, such as static contraction of the muscles—working muscles against the force of other muscles—which when practised regularly keep the muscles in good trim. Such exercises as dips or press-ups, done in various ways, are resistance exercises, for the body weight provides the resistance. This particular exercise in its many forms is one of the best resistance exercises known, and it appears in many of the exercise schedules in this book. Here are one or two self-resistance exercises you may like to try:

Sitting on a chair, extend each thigh alternately and tightly contract the thigh muscles, hold the contraction for three or four seconds, and then relax. Repeat several times each thigh.

With chair support, rise on the toes as far as possible, contract the calf vigorously, hold for three or four seconds and relax. Repeat several times each leg, separately and together.

Clench the fist tightly and bend the arm completely contracting the biceps, hold for three or four seconds and repeat each arm. This exercise can be done by bending both arms and pressing the cupped hands against each other so contracting the biceps. Tightly clenching and unclenching the fist, will work the muscles of the forearm.

Another form of resistance exercise for the upper arm is to flex the arm and place the flat of the hand at the back of one's neck, and then contract the biceps muscles.

Back lying, breathe out slowly and raise the head, contracting the abdominal muscles tightly. This can also be done standing.

Stand close to a table and push with the flat of the hand against it. Do the same with arms extended and push against a wall.

Hold the arms above the head fingers hooked, pull outwards and downwards for shoulder and upper arm effect.

Hook the fingers in front of the chest and push and pull. This is a good strengthener for the chest muscles.

Later in this book I have given some good resistance exercises to be done with two people using a towel or even a piece of rope.

The main purposes of such exercises by contracting the muscles is for strengthening. The great drawback is that resistance cannot be carefully graduated in these self-applied exercises, and while the muscles used gain in strength and suppleness they do not increase in shape and size as quickly as they do when graduated resistance with apparatus is applied.

CHAPTER EIGHT

A Gym at Home

Many people make the excuse that they cannot do any form of training because lack of time or distance, prevent them from attending a club or gym. Others have no club facilities nearby. Many are students or young fellows with little cash to spend on expensive equipment. Where there is a real desire to do some form of progressive resistance work, it is amazing what can be done with a little initiative and ingenuity.

The purpose of this chapter is to try to give you a few ideas about a make-do gym which you can adapt to your own use and circumstances. The first requirement is space. You may be lucky enough to have a spare room, a garage or a shed which you can transform by degrees into a little gym and possibily get a couple of friends to train with you. Or you can perhaps use the box-room or attic. But the majority of people have only their bedroom or a small bed-sitting-room.

Some consideration will naturally have to be given to the size of your training space and whether you are situated in an upper room, ground floor, or anywhere where any too-vigorous form of exercise might disturb others, or upset a touchy landlady. You don't want to risk bringing a ceiling down, or making cracks in the roof of an old house, by jumping about too much. If you are a downstairs tenant, you rightly get annoyed when your neighbours disturb the peace! Even the freestanding exercises in the previous chapter may have to be modified according to your

A Gym at Home

facilities. You may find it quite impracticable to do some of the upward jumping or leg movements unless you are particularly light on your feet.

Generally speaking, there is ample room, even in a small bed-sitting-room, to do all the freestanding exercises I have suggested with little inconvenience to anyone.

Provided you have room to swing your arms freely, and to lie full length on the floor for abdominal work, you can almost cover your requirements. You can take it, therefore, that a space of 8 ft. x 7 ft. or even less would give you sufficient room to carry out a full exercise routine.

If you are exercising in your own room, make sure there is adequate ventilation. This does not necessarily mean a draught, but do ensure a reasonable flow of fresh air. Exercising in a warm fuggy room is only fatiguing, and much of the benefit is lost. If you have any heating like a gas fire that you can turn off during exercise, do so, but do not sit about catching cold. In cold weather wear loose warm clothing for exercise.

Most rooms have some pieces of furniture which can be used for resistance work. For instance, with feet on the bed or an upright chair, and hands on the arms of a fireside or armchair, you have an excellent base for dips, which is an excellent arm, shoulder and chest exercise. This, and others suggested, were described in the previous chapter.

A heavy book like an encyclopaedia can be used for a great variety of exercises. These come to mind quickly: pull over a arms' length, taking the book to thighs; single arm presses; single arm curls; single arm swings. If two books are available to the above can be added lateral raise sideways and upwards alternate forward and upward swings and side bends.

If you can get a small plank of wood about 3 ft. long and 12 to 18 inches wide, you can improvise a little bench by standing the plank on a couple of books, and covering it with an old blanket or cloth.

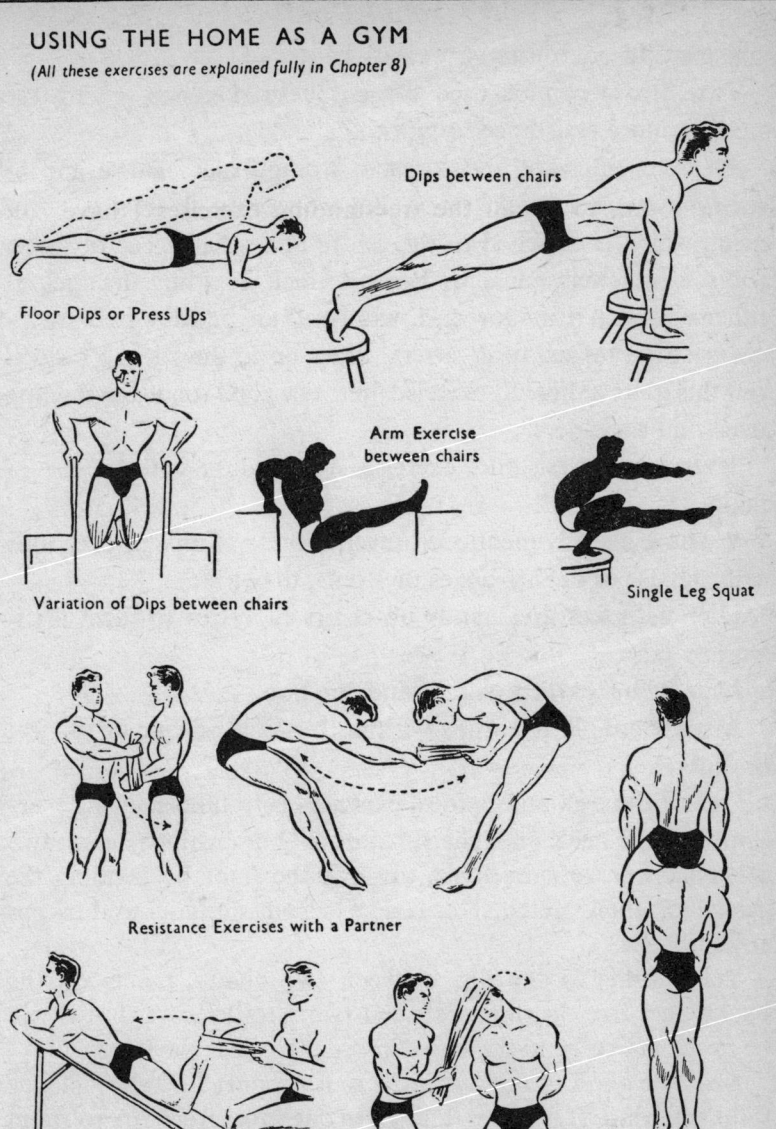

USING THE HOME AS A GYM

(All these exercises are explained fully in Chapter 8)

Dips between chairs

Floor Dips or Press Ups

Arm Exercise between chairs

Variation of Dips between chairs

Single Leg Squat

Resistance Exercises with a Partner

A piece of board can very easily be stored.

Two bricks can be used for all these exercises, giving the muscles more resistance to work against.

An excellent wrist and forearm strengthener can be improvised by tying a brick, stone, flat iron or book to a piece of string which is attached to the centre of a small piece of wood about a foot long and 1 to 2 inches thick. Holding the stick at either end with arms forward, wind and unwind the string with the weight attached to it, several times on to the stick. You will find this quite a difficult exercise, but very good for strengthening arms and shoulders.

Several good resistance exercises can be done with the use of chairs.

We have already mentioned several forms of dips or press ups with the use of chairs, boxes or stools, they are:

Dips with feet and hands on chairs or boxes to form a triangular base.

Dips with feet on a chair, hands on floor.

A more simple one, dips with both hands on one chair, feet on floor.

One of the best and hardest exercises is to take a sitting position with the heels on a chair, hands slightly behind you on two others, lower your buttocks towards the floor by bending the arms, and then stretch. This is an excellent shoulder and triceps strengthener.

Yet another is the dip between two chairs, hands on the backs, feet free, as done between two parallel bars, but it will be necessary to bend the knees in order to clear the floor.

Another good use of a chair is as a support for the single leg full knee bend. It is better, and gives one more freedom, to stand on the chair seat on one leg, with the other leg forward. Holding on the back of the chair with one hand try doing a full knee bend and stretch. Turn to support with other hand and repeat with the other leg. This is a very strong exercise for the quadriceps of the thigh and the knee joint.

A Gym at Home

If you are lucky enough to be in your own home, you can purchase an adjustable bar which fits in any doorway, and can be put up or removed in a matter of seconds without any fear of damaging the woodwork. On this you can not only do many forms of pull ups, or 'chinning' as we call it, but it is also ideal for abdominal work such as legs raise and knees raise.

Chinning or pull ups can be done in several ways, overgrasp, under grasp, and the pull up to behind the neck position, if space permits.

By putting this bar low to the floor, you can do certain exercises that are usually done on a beam such as back hanging grasping the bar, pull to chest. Sitting on floor, pull to chest by lifting hips off floor. Details of chinning exercises are given in a later chapter.

If you are able to fit hooks to the wainscot in your room various types of expander work for legs, abdominals, etc., can be done.

There are several types of expander on the market that have the necessary fittings to adapt them for leg and abdominal work. Something combined of this kind is better for all-round work than the simple straightforward 'chest' expander.

In Chapter Nine, I give you some suggested exercises for expanders.

Provided that you are free to jump about as much as you please, all forms of skipping are ideal for speed, stamina, and co-ordination. Skipping is a much neglected form of exercise, but done correctly has considerable effect on heart, lungs and circulation.

A medicine ball, even if one trains alone, is a useful added form of resistance, particularly for abdominal work. For example:

1. Back lying, arms above the head holding a medicine ball, trunk raise to forward reach, to touch the head on knees, and the medicine ball at the feet.

2. Back lying, ball held between feet, raise legs holding ball.

3. Back lying, place ball behind head. Legs raise to touch floor behind head, and pick ball up.

4. Place the ball on the floor, and roll on it with the abdomen. This is an old toughening and reducing exercise often employed by boxers.

5. Ball held at arms' length overhead, trunk circling.

6. *Trunk exercises.* A good trunk movement is to hold the ball at arms' length feet astride, trunk relaxed bending down to swing the ball between the legs, and return to upright.

7. Stand astride, hold ball above head. Trunk bend freely from side to side.

8. Hold the ball in front of your waist, move ball from left to right with trunk twisting, trying to keep hips square to front.

9. If space permits—single arm throwing upwards with medicine ball, or even single arm presses.

10. Stand astride, hold ball at arms' length, drop arms behind head holding the ball and stretch them to upright.

These are just a few of the many exercises that can be done single handed with a medicine ball. If there are two of you training together you can include the many forms of throwing, twisting, catching, etc., and the scope is greatly widened.

ISOMETRICS

A fairly modern form of self resistance is styled as *Isometrics*, but really it is a modernized version of self-resistance. Pressing against a wall with one or both hands would be an isometric exercise, as would clasping the hands together and trying to pull them apart.

Like all new 'gimmicks' Isometrics found a place in the keep-fit vocabulary.

Some athletes use this form of exercise very successfully, for added strength. Several appliances have appeared on the market, and one which will improve back strength is a chain, against which you pull, fastened to a platform and with a dial to register the poundage you are pulling.

Another is to fix a bar on stands so that it is immovable, and a lifter endeavours to press it overhead, so using the muscles involved in this particular form of exercise.

A great many exercises can be devised which would come under the heading of Isometrics.

GADGETS AND GIMMICKS

There are always new gadgets and gimmicks on the market, many with terrific advertising campaigns to launch them and excellent PR people to handle them.

I am always being asked what I think of some new appliance, and it is hard to comment.

To begin with people are always looking for 'an easy way' and when claims are made that a new gadget will give you fitness, strength and a physique in half the time of weight training, then there will always be a ready market of people to try it out.

My humble opinion is that there is no substitute for weight training, but that any gadget that induces someone to take stock of their fitness and health is well worth while.

However, try not to get too carried away with the fantastic claims; the power of advertising is amazing!

CHAPTER NINE

How to Use the Equipment

I n recent years there has been a terrific advance in the manufacture of all kinds of new equipment. Anyone visiting a really modern health studio will be amazed at the vast array of expensive-looking benches, incline benches, abdominal boards, pulleys and 'jungle pulleys' of all shapes and sizes, thigh extension, leg press and calf machines, vibrators, gym cycles, etc. But fundamentally, and coming down to brass tacks, they are only more attractive editions of the basic barbell and dumbbells, bench, squat stands and pulley. However, they are certainly a psychological inducement to attract more customers and make training a more enjoyable and less boring chore.

Many young bodybuilders meet with difficulty in finding a suitable form of equipment to provide progressive resistance. Many others prefer to use more than one type of equipment.

EXPANDERS

Expanders offer a very useful form of resistance training with a wide range of exercises. They are very handy to carry about, need little space for packing, and are light. This makes them very useful for the traveller and for the home-trainer.

There are several different types of expanders, and all have their merits. They also have a variety of names according to what they are made of. They are called: SPRINGS, CABLES, STRANDS, or CHEST EXPANDERS or as 'combination' outfits under various trade names.

76

They are made of steel springs, rubber, or strands of elastic covered with a fabric.

Steel strands, though normally lasting for years, can be over-stretched with misuse, and are liable to pinch the skin when exercises are done with the springs near the body, if care is not taken. Plain or solid rubber is rather inclined to crack in time and become perished if not kept in good condition, while fabric covered ones also deteriorate if used in a faulty manner. Nowadays both springs and elastic-cord strands are made of different lengths to suit the reach of the purchaser, while most springs have check cords to prevent them being too far extended.

The other slight drawback of Expanders is that increases in resistance can only be made by adding another strand or spring. These increases usually jump in the nature of 10 lb., which is rather a big increase in some exercises.

However, one of the great advantages of expander work, is that it maintains a wonderful mobility of muscles and joints, and promotes strength in tendons and ligaments.

As I told you earlier, there are various fittings available which adapt expanders for doing leg and other exercises, so that the scope is widened.

Here are a few suggested exercises for the expanders. Like weight training, I suggest that you try the SET SYSTEM, doing each exercise for two, three or four sets of repetitions as required, with a rest between each set.

1. Single Arm Front Chest Pull

This is one of the first exercises to learn. Stand astride or feet together, holding the expander, one arm out sideways, palm to front, and the other hand knuckles forward across the chest. Keeping one arm straight out sideways, pull the expander across chest with the other arm, until both arms are in line. Repeat several repetitions, then change to opposite side.

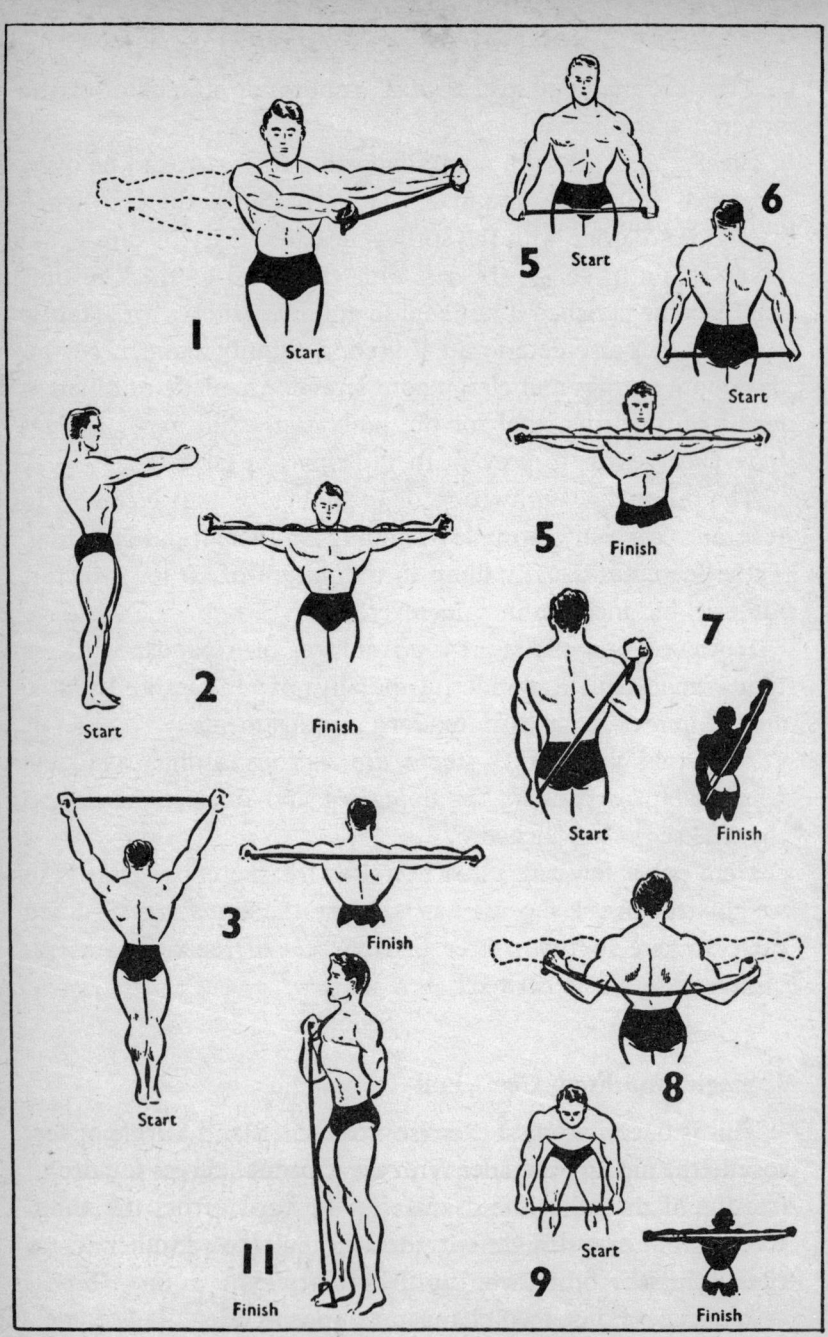

A FEW SIMPLE EXPANDER EXERCISES

How to Use the Equipment

2. Two Hands Front Chest Pull

Stand astride or feet together, hold the expander at arms' length in front, knuckles outward. Keeping the arms straight pull the expander until the strands touch the chest. This exercise can also be done palms outwards, but is not quite so effective. This is a good back and chest exercise.

3. Overhead Downward Pull

Stand astride or feet together, holding an expander at arms' length above the head, palms outwards. Keeping arms straight pull expander downwards across the chest or behind the neck. This is a fine latissimus, triceps and chest exercise.

4. Overhead Downward Pull Palms Inward

This is the same as the above exercise, but a little more difficult.

5. Front Lateral Raise

Stand astride or feet together holding an expander in front of the thighs knuckles outwards. Keeping the expander close to the body, raise the arms sideways. This is very strong deltoid and pectoral exercise.

6. Back Lateral Raise

The same exercise as above, but commencing with the expanders held across the back of the buttocks. This is also a deltoid exercise, but affects the latissimus and back.

7. Single Arm Press

Stand feet astride or together, one hand holding the expander close to the hip at your side. With the expander across the back, hold the other end at the shoulder, palm to the front. Keeping lower arm still at side, extend the other arm overhead. Repeat several times, and then change to opposite side.

This is a good deltoid, triceps and general shoulder exercise.

8. Two Hands Back Press

Stand feet together or astride. Hold the expander across the centre of the back knuckles outwards. Stretch both arms out sideways finishing with the expander across the shoulders.

This is a good back and arm exercise.

9. Bent Forward Front Chest Pull

Stand astride holding the expander knuckles outwards with arms in the hang position. Bend forward so that the body is at right angles to the legs. Maintaining the forward bend position, stretch the expanders across the chest. This is a strong chest, shoulder and arm exercise.

10. Single Arm Curl (illustration 11)

Hold one end of the expander with the foot in the handle, toes on the floor to prevent handle slipping. Stand erect with the other hand palm upward under the other handle. Curl the arm by flexing the upper arm, until the expander is near the chin. This is a fine upper arm exercise. Repeat with each arm.

11. Reverse Curl

The same as the curl, but knuckles are uppermost, and the handle is gripped from the top. This is a strong exercise for the forearm muscles.

12. Single Arm Rowing (Not illustrated.)

Holding one end of the expander under the foot, other end held knuckles upward in front of the body. Pull the expander upwards towards the chest by flexing the elbow outwards, and not as above where the upper arm is kept stationary at the side.

All these exercises can of course be done in varying positions for more scope. For instance the FRONT CHEST PULL can be done lying down. Many of them can be done seated for added progression, such as the OVERHEAD DOWNWARD PULL. Others can be combined with freestanding movements, such as SQUATS combined with FRONT CHEST PULL.

By fixing attachments to a wall, or getting special stirrups, you can do such exercises as THIGH EXTENSIONS sitting on a chair, PULLOVERS and various abdominal exercises on the floor.

Expander work can also be used with such exercises as dips or press ups with feet and hands on chairs or boxes. Assuming that you have a set of expanders, here is a little schedule you may like to try.

General loosening up with freestanding exercises, then:

SINGLE ARM PRESS (Ex. 7). 2 sets of 10 repetitions each arm.

OVERHEAD DOWNWARD PULL (Ex. 3). 2 sets of 10 repetitions.

SINGLE ARM CURL (Ex. 10). 3 sets of 8 repetitions each arm.

FRONT LATERAL RAISE (Ex. 5). 2 sets of 10 repetitions.

SIT UPS performing FRONT CHEST PULL (Ex. 2). 2 sets of 12 repetitions.

SINGLE LEG SQUATS with support. 2 sets of 10 repetitions each leg.

SIDE BENDS. Holding expander outstretched across shoulders, and feet astride—trunk bend side to side to count of 30.

DIPS or Press ups with feet and hands on chairs or boxes 3 sets of 10 repetitions.

Use one or two strands as required, but ensure that all exercises are done CORRECTLY.

WALL BARS (illustration page 89)

Many physical culture studios, clubs and gymnasia have wall bars fixed, and though they are greatly neglected by bodybuilders we think they are invaluable for certain types of exercises to promote mobility and suppleness, and especially for remedial purposes. But for the bodybuilder their main value is in two or three excellent abdominal exercises not possible on other apparatus, and also for some good lateral work.

The type of bars I refer to are those which look like a ladder fastened to the wall, and with rungs about a foot apart. Here are one or two simple exercises you may like to try if you are fortunate to train in a place that has wall bars.

ALTERNATE KNEE RAISE: Stand with back against the wall bars arms above the head grasping the nearest bar so that you are reaching up at arms' length and supporting your weight Alternate knee raise high to chest.

BACK HANGING KNEES RAISE: Back hang from the top wall bar. Both knees raise high to chest. Lower and repeat. This is an excellent more-advanced exercise for the lower abdomen. Try and reach 3 sets of 10 repetitions.

BACK HANGING LEGS RAISE: Back hanging from the top wall bar. Both legs raise to right angles with body. This is a very advanced and excellent abdominal exercise. Both these exercises can of course also be done on a chinning bar, but are not so effective as the absence of back rest creates difficulty in controlling the swinging motion which develops.

SIDE STANDING TRUNK BENDING SIDEWAYS: Stand sideways to the wall bars with one leg extended and supported on about the fifth rung of the wall bars. Hands on hips or neck rest, trunk bend side to side towards and away from the wall bars, keeping body straight. Progression to this exercise is to raise the leg supported against the wall bars to a higher rung, until the leg is at right angles to the trunk.

FORWARD LEG SUPPORT TRUNK BEND FORWARD: The same exercise as above can be done by placing the leg straight into the fifth rung, and then bending the trunk towards the forward leg.

How to Use the Equipment

This is an excellent exercise for those with short hamstrings, and the progression is to raise the leg on a higher rung until it is at right angles to the trunk. Rear leg must be kept straight.

WALL EXERCISERS

There are several types of pulleys and wall exercisers fastened to the wall, and you may see these in a well-equipped club. They are used for remedial purposes, and offer quite a wide scope of special exercises. Some are of the double handled type so that each arm can be exercised separately, others have but one handle. This type of wall exerciser has so many variations that to try and enumerate the exercises would be impossible within the scope of this book. It can be used for downward pulls, upward pulls, single arm curls, pullovers, etc., in lying, seated or standing position.

The most popular type of pulley you will find in bodybuilding clubs now is the overhead type suspended from the ceiling with a handle at one end of the wire and a rod at the other to which weights can be added or subtracted, thus offering a wide range of resistance.

As this type of overhead pulley is so widely used, I will outline a few exercises for this type of apparatus.

OVERHEAD PULLEY (illustration page 85)

This type of pulley is often fitted with a straight handle, but it is better to use one with a curved bar to fit across the shoulders when pulled down. It is excellent for a beginner, particularly one with stiff shoulders, protruding shoulder blades, or a stoop.

Remember that as most of the exercises can be done STANDING, SEATED or even LYING, I will not repeat them in each different position. I prefer most of the exercises to be done in a kneeling position, keeping the trunk erect without sag. Exercises are done on the SET SYSTEM.

How to Use the Equipment

1. Pull to Chest

For better range of movement do this kneeling or sitting on a stool. Grasp the handle of the pulley one hand each side of the pulley bar, and pull to chest. This is a fine deltoid, and latissimus exercise. 50 lb. would make a good starting poundage.

2. Pull Behind Neck

This is about the finest and most widely used pulley exercise. Kneeling or sitting, grasp the pulley handles, and pull the handles to touch the nape of the neck. This is a wonderful shoulder, latissimus, and arm exercise, and ideal for poor posture. We suggest that 40 lb. would make a good trial.

3. Narrow Reverse Grip Downward Pull

Kneeling or sitting as before, grasp the handles of the pulley, narrow grip under grasp. Pull the bar down to the chest using the biceps. This is a fine biceps exercise. Try 40 lb.

4. Triceps Stretch

Stand close to the pulley. With narrow grip, hands placed on top of handle, press the pulley downwards until the arms are extended downwards to the thighs. This is a fine exercise for the triceps, and a tough one. Try with 30 lb.

5. Back Lying on a Bench Pull to Chest

Lie with your head towards the pulley. Grasp the handle at arms' length, and pull the handle to the chest. This is a fine chest exercise. Try with 50 lb. for a start.

6. Back Lying Curl

The same exercise as above, but grasp the pulley undergrasp narrow grip, and pull the handle to the chest by flexing the forearms.

These are but a few of the well-known exercises for an over-

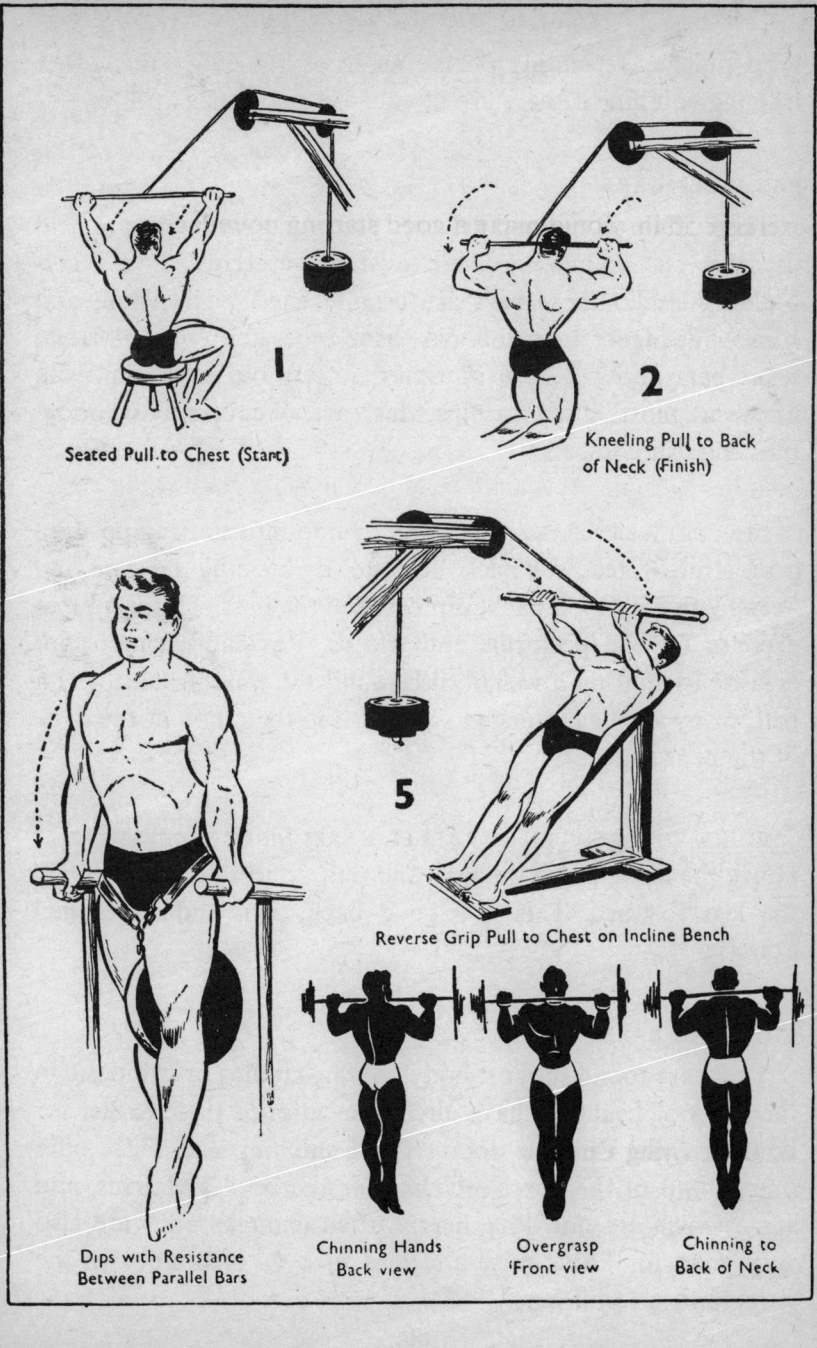

1. Seated Pull to Chest (Start)

2. Kneeling Pull to Back of Neck (Finish)

5. Reverse Grip Pull to Chest on Incline Bench

Dips with Resistance Between Parallel Bars

Chinning Hands Back view

Overgrasp Front view

Chinning to Back of Neck

head pulley. Depending on the angle of the pulley and other training equipment there are of course a great many more.

PARALLEL BARS

The ordinary type parallel bars used for gymnastics are also used for one or two excellent resistance exercises. In a body-building studio these bars are usually fixed to the wall, and somewhat higher than the gymnastic type, and consist of two short bars about 2 ft. 6 in. apart, jutting out from the wall. These are mostly used for dips which are, of course, basic body-building exercises.

DIPS BETWEEN PARALLEL BARS: Jump into starting position arms straight, feet well back, head up. By bending the arms and keeping the feet well back, dip between the bars. This is a great exercise for the pectorals and triceps. Resistance can be increased by putting a weight disc round the waist fastened by a belt, or by holding a loaded swing bell in the crook at the back of the bent knees.

PULLS UP BETWEEN PARALLEL BARS: Sit on the floor, arms above the head, grasp the bars and pull up to the chest keeping the legs forward. This is a good back, arm and abdominal exercise.

CHINNING BARS

These are found in most bodybuilding studios or gymnasia in the form of beams. I have already mentioned them earlier for home training with the door type of chinning bar. These offer one or two of the finest exercises for the back and arms, and some which are not done nearly often enough. They are also very good for knees raise and legs raise as mentioned in the paragraph on wall bars.

How to Use the Equipment

The three main back and arm exercises are as follows:

CHINNING OR PULL UPS OVERGRASP: Jump on to the bar with hands overgrasp, knuckles uppermost, hands slightly wider than shoulder width apart. Keeping the heels well back and with no forward body movements or jerking, pull up until the chest touches the bar, and lower. If you can do three sets of 8 or 10 repetitions in this exercise, you are doing very well. Resistance can be added as in the parallel bar dips, by adding weight round the waist or in the crook behind the bent knees.

CHINNING TO BACK OF NECK: This is the same exercise as above, but more advanced. Instead of pulling to the chest, pull until the back of the neck touches the bar. Both these are wonderful exercises particularly for the latissimus muscles, and for the whole back.

CHINNING UNDERGRASP: The position is the same as for the other two exercises, but the grip is narrower and the palms face you instead of being away from you. This exercise puts more work on the arms than the other exercises.

IRON BOOTS

These are a type of iron shoe which you wear strapped over your training shoes or boots. They weigh around 8 lb. each, and underneath have a groove where you can insert a short dumbell rod to take discs for extra weight and resistance. They are used mostly for leg and abdominal work, and offer a wide scope for those seeking extra powerful leg muscles and muscular separation, and for minor remedial purposes. The poundage added depends on the individual. At first it will be quite enough to try the exercises without any added weight.

How to Use the Equipment

LEG EXERCISES

1. Sitting Thigh Extension

Sit on a table or chair, legs at the hang. Straighten alternate knee, at the same time flexing the quadriceps muscles. This is a fine quadriceps exercise, and also a strengthener for the knee joint, and in a modified way is extensively used by footballers, etc., in the treatment of knee injuries. As a leg builder, you will need some extra weight right from the start. Try with an added 10 lb. to the weight of the boot. Some top-flight footballers can use a 100 lb. in this exercise!

2. Standing Alternate Leg Raise

Alternate leg raise to right angles with body. This is also a special quadriceps and general thigh exercise.

3. Standing Alternate Leg Swings

As above, but swing the leg forward and backward. This is a fine hip and buttock exercise.

4. Standing Back Curl

With support and with some added weight on the boots, bend the leg backwards from the knee, contracting the calf muscle. This is a fine exercise. Try high repetitions with each leg about a set of 15 each side, and add 10 lb. to the weight of the boot.

5. Standing Leg Raise Sideways

With support, alternate leg raise sideways from the hip. This is a fine hip exercise, and also for the muscles on the inside of the leg, and the oblique muscles of the abdomen.

Certain light jumping exercises can also be done wearing the boots (without weights) provided the floor is strong enough and noise doesn't matter.

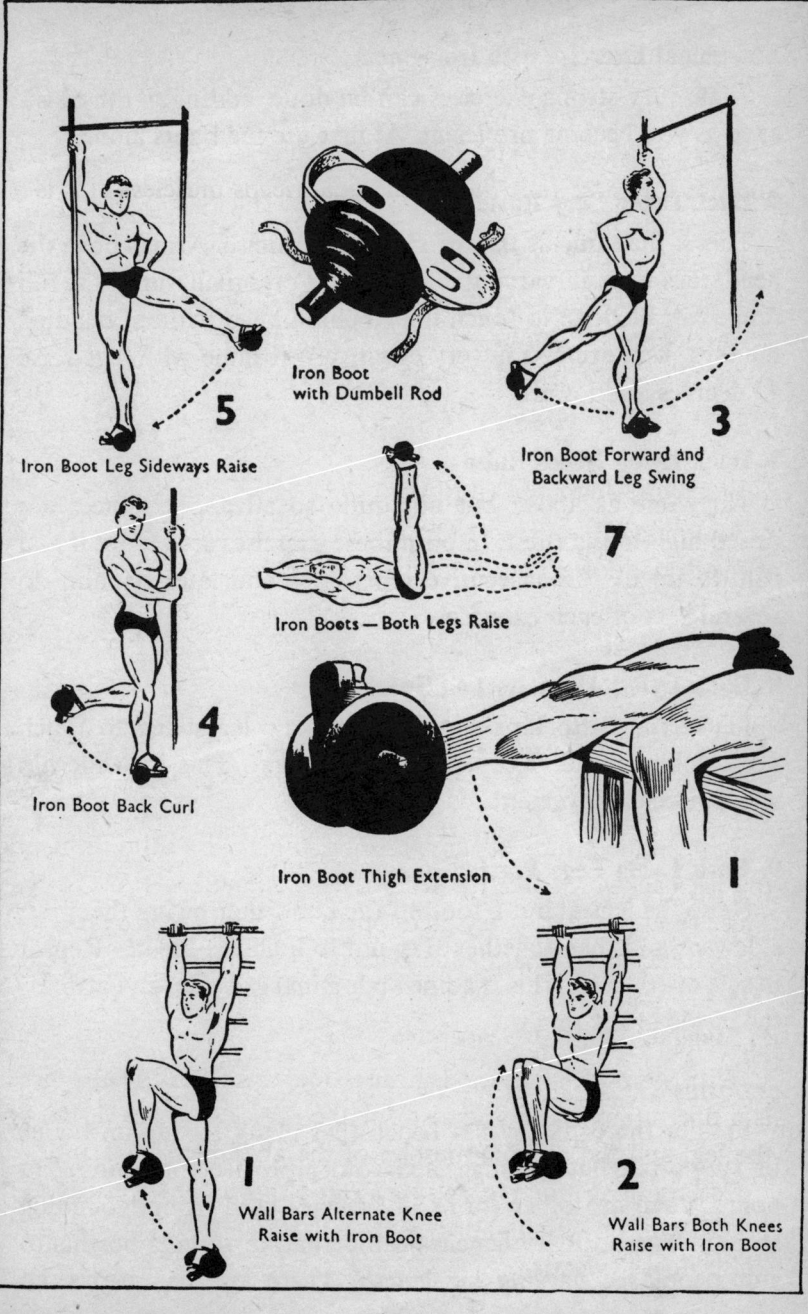

Iron Boot
with Dumbell Rod

Iron Boot Leg Sideways Raise

5

Iron Boot Forward and
Backward Leg Swing

3

7

Iron Boots — Both Legs Raise

Iron Boot Back Curl

4

Iron Boot Thigh Extension

1

Wall Bars Alternate Knee
Raise with Iron Boot

1

Wall Bars Both Knees
Raise with Iron Boot

2

Abdominal Exercise with Iron Boots

Some very strong exercises can be done, adding to the resistance as you become proficient. At first use the boots alone.

6. Back Lying Legs Raise

This is the same as the freestanding exercise. Arms above the head, legs raise in varying degrees, and eventually until the full range can be done to touch floor behind head without bending the legs. The exercise is very effective just done with legs raise 45 degrees and lower.

7. Back Lying Knees Raise

The same as above but not quite so advanced. Knees are raised high to the chest. In both these exercises see at first if you can do up to 10 consecutive repetitions and later try and do several sets of each exercise.

8. Back Lying Alternate Leg Swing

Back lying with hips support, alternate leg swing to touch floor behind head. Keep both legs straight. This is a fine hip and buttocks movement.

9. Back Lying Legs Parting

Raise the legs about a foot off the floor, then swing them out sideways and then together. Try not to hold the breath. Repeat in sets of 10 to 15. This is a fine abdominal exercise, and also for the inside of the thighs.

BENCHES

Besides the ordinary flat bench (flat plank resting on books or supports) that we suggested you improvise for training at home, there are other forms of benches used in bodybuilding studios. The ordinary benches can be had in varying heights to suit people of varying leg length. There are also INCLINED

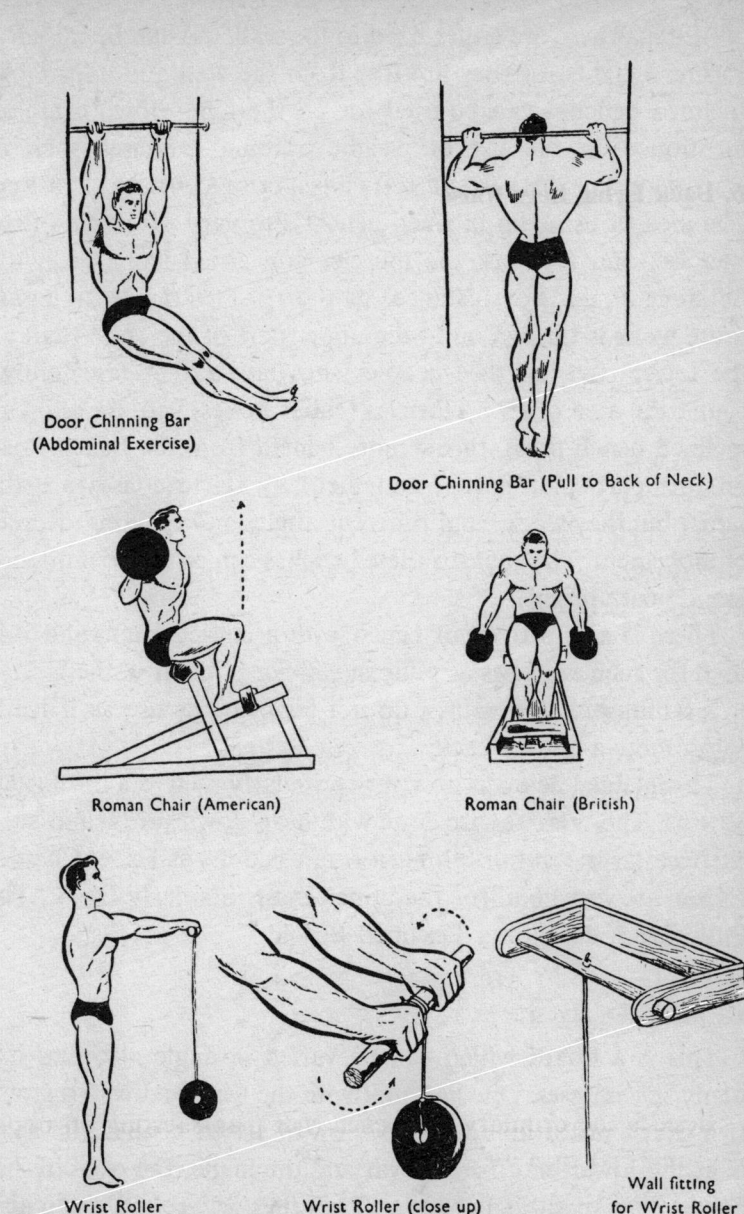

Door Chinning Bar
(Abdominal Exercise)

Door Chinning Bar (Pull to Back of Neck)

Roman Chair (American)

Roman Chair (British)

Wrist Roller

Wrist Roller (close up)

Wall fitting
for Wrist Roller

BENCHES. These are either fixed to the wall and can be raised to various heights, or they are free from the wall and adjustable. Inclined benches can be used for all the lying down exercises mentioned in the list of weight training exercises such as BENCH PRESS, DUMBELL BENCH PRESS, CURLS, PULLOVERS, ETC. The idea of using an inclined bench is to vary the angle of the exercise, and so work the muscles concerned from a slightly different angle. For instance, in the INCLINED BENCH PRESS more work is thrown on to the upper part of the chest than on the lower part, so that people who have rather big hollows round the area of their clavicles (collar bones) can, by using an inclined bench press, throw more benefit from the Bench Press on this particular part. Fundamentally the exercises are the same, but they work from different angles and different degrees of movement. The angle of these benches can be varied until they are almost upright.

There is also a form of bench with a curved back, and it is used for such exercises as pullovers. Once popular in the U.S.A. it is falling out of favour. I do not advocate its use as it tends to promote a hollow back.

The inclined bench is now very popularly used as a DECLINED BENCH. The exercises are done with head downwards, and such exercises as the DECLINED BENCH PRESS done as Ex. 6, Chapter Eleven are very good for the upper chest. Similarly Ex. 4., The Pullover, is done on a Declined Bench.

ABDOMINAL BOARD

This is a board which can be varied in angle also and has many special uses. One lies on it with the feet fixed with a strap. It it excellent for an advanced form of SIT UPS, when the head is at the lower end, for, by varying the angle, the exercise becomes correspondingly harder. The other way round it can also be used for legs raise.

How to Use the Equipment

CALF EXERCISE MACHINE

In some clubs you will find also a piece of apparatus specially designed for lower leg work. It takes the form of a harness with two rods to put across your shoulder and a chain. With toes on a block of wood, you can perform heels raising on this and give the calves a strong work out. Additional weight is easily put on to the harness.

LEG PRESSING MACHINE

There are various types of apparatus for heavy leg work but generally they comprise a platform which holds the weights, under which you can lie and press the weights up and down. It is a favourite exercise of racing cyclists who build massive leg strength with this apparatus.

ROMAN CHAIR

This is another modern gadget for special leg work. It is simple to construct, and gives exceptionally fine leg exercises. The simplicity of it is that exercises can be done without apparatus using the body weight as resistance, or with weights.

There are, of course, many other training gadgets which have their particular merit. Of these, perhaps two others are of interest.

HEAD HARNESS

This, as the name implies, is a strap affair which fits on the head and its special purpose is for neck strengthening exercises. Weights are added to the special fitting and increased as the exerciser requires. Here are two basic neck developers.

KNEELING ON CHAIR OR TABLE. Head raise and lower.

BACK LYING, NECK DROP AND LIFT OVER END OF BENCH
It is a useful piece of equipment though the normal exercises

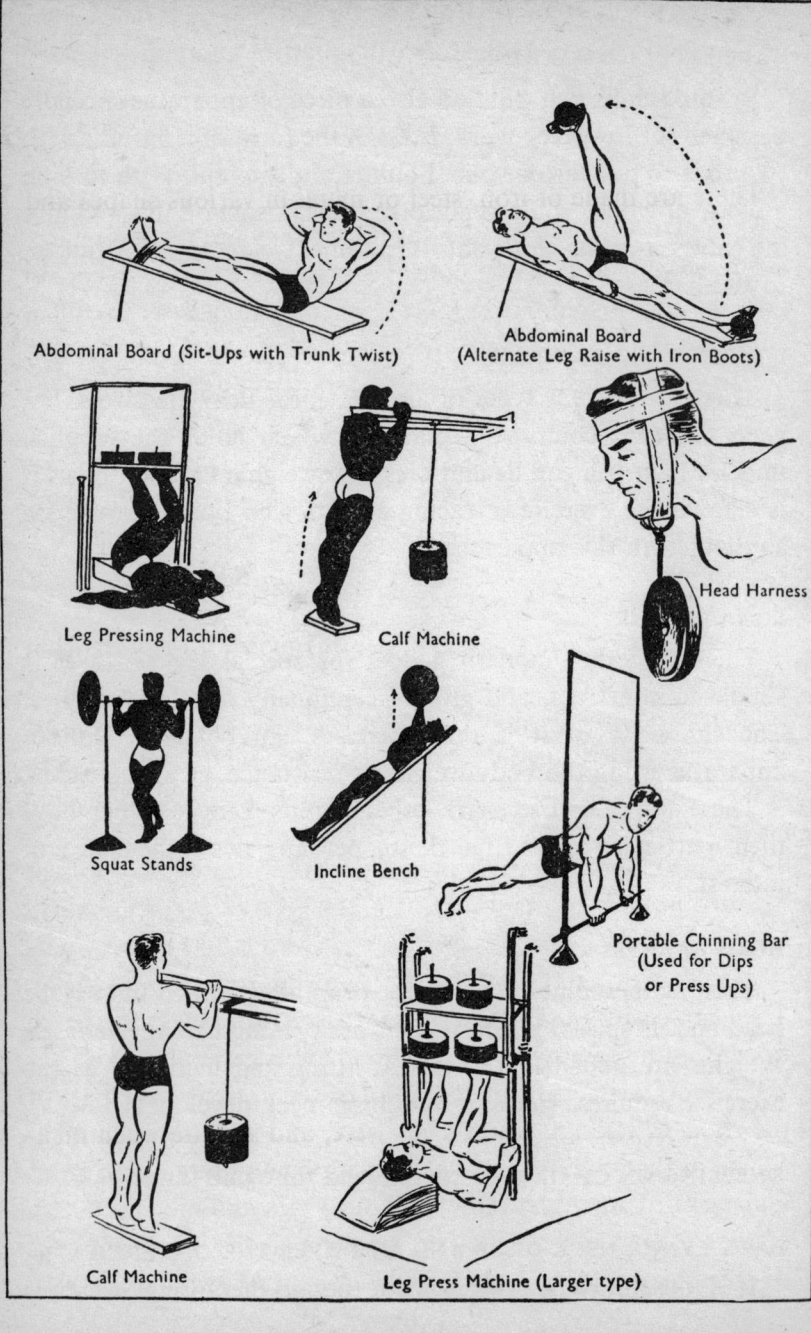

Abdominal Board (Sit-Ups with Trunk Twist)

Abdominal Board (Alternate Leg Raise with Iron Boots)

Leg Pressing Machine

Calf Machine

Head Harness

Squat Stands

Incline Bench

Portable Chinning Bar (Used for Dips or Press Ups)

Calf Machine

Leg Press Machine (Larger type)

of a properly planned schedule will all affect and improve neck strength and shape.

SQUAT STANDS

These are made of iron, steel or metal in various shapes and sizes, some fixed and some adjustable. They are made to carry heavy weights at a height convenient to the exerciser who can take the weights at shoulder level when he could not lift them from the floor. They enable heavy weights to be used for the Squats which form a basic part of most body building programmes.

They can also be adjusted to use with the Bench Press exercise (Ex. 6, page 109) and are very useful when exercising alone or with one training partner.

SAUNA BATHS

The Sauna bath has largely taken the place of the old steam and Turkish baths and steam cabinets. No modern health studio is complete to-day without a Sauna bath. In fact, it is probably the most lucrative health-giving asset of a modern health studio. It is less messy than a steam bath and far easier to run and keep clean.

There are many types, in many sizes; they can be built to seat up to fifteen or more people at a time, or they can be small enough to install in a private house, and many house-owners who can afford this modern health-giving luxury have them. They can cost thousands or a hundred or two, and can even be bought on hire purchase. There are many reputable makes.

They originated in Finland and for generations were part of the ritual of taking a bath. They were, and still are when mentioned in that country, associated with being beaten with twigs and even rolling in the snow! But in Britain and modern health studios they have merely taken the place of the old steam bath or steam cabinets, and are very beneficial to health.

How to Use the Equipment

To-day, hardworking executives and business-women find a Sauna a natural way of relaxing and improving and preserving their physique or figure.

The human body, by perspiring and eliminating all the toxins, is performing a natural function.

Young and old may participate in a Sauna and then, if they wish, relish the cooling feeling of a shower afterwards.

They are not really expensive to run and are very easy to take care of.

CHAPTER TEN

Training with Weights at Home

One of the most remarkable facts of Modern Body-building is that the manufacturers of weightlifting appliances are doing an ever increasing business not only in providing clubs and gymnasia with all kinds of heavy weightlifting outfits but in supplying thousands of home training sets to individuals every year. This is in itself practical proof that home training with weights is popular. No matter how many clubs and barbell studios are open there are always persons who prefer to train on their own. And they do achieve splendid results.

Now I feel it necessary to treat the reader as a beginner who, having become convinced of the need to train at home, wonders how to go about it.

First let me say that you don't need much space. You can train at home without much interference to your family. You needn't make much noise and you won't damage the furniture. And remember you can do sufficient training in as little as fifteen minutes two or three times a week to attain health and fitness, though if you want strength and increased muscular development this will take longer.

Now a word about appliances:

APPLIANCES

Weight-training or Barbell sets usually comprise a steel bar of 1 inch in diameter in varying lengths from 4 ft. to 6 ft. Most sets also include two dumbell rods of 18 inches in length with a sleeve, which revolves, and four collars with screws or patent bolts for securing the weights to the bar or dumbells. The weights are made up of discs of different sizes and vary from 3 inches upwards in diameter. The discs themselves can be from 50 lb. each to 1¼ lb. in weight and are made of cast iron.

The weights required for a complete beginner really depend on your purse and also your ultimate aims. Weight-training equipment is fairly expensive, but remember that it lasts a lifetime, also that if you can only afford a very light set to commence with, you can always add more weight to it as means become available, and also as you progress. Your initial strength must be taken into consideration as well.

If you can afford it, I recommend that the set you get should include a barbell as well as dumbell rods, as this will greatly widen the scope of your exercises, but in case you cannot, we will include one or two suggested schedules for a barbell only, for dumbells only, and for combined work.

The only additional equipment you will really need is an improvised bench or form, unless of course you are fortunate enough to be able to set yourself up really well with all sorts of extra appliances which are available. In this chapter I will deal with the bare necessities, and suggest how you can best utilize them.

An ordinary form will be ideal for the bench, but if not available, a plank of wood 2 ft. 6 in. to 3 ft. in length, and 1 ft. to 1 ft. 6 in. wide, would suit your purpose admirably. You can improvise a bench by standing it on two further blocks of wood or logs, or even big books, so that it is not less than a foot high, and not more than 2 feet high. This will be needed for many of the lying down exercises, in which you lie with feet either side of the bench with feet firmly on the floor. An old piece of blanket put on the bench will give added comfort.

If you can only afford a 50–90 lb. set of weights for a start, it will have to do (and is really ample, for most) except for two exercises known as The Squat or Knees Bend for the legs, and the Bench Press for shoulders and chest, at which even a complete beginner would begin at about 50 lb., and would very soon

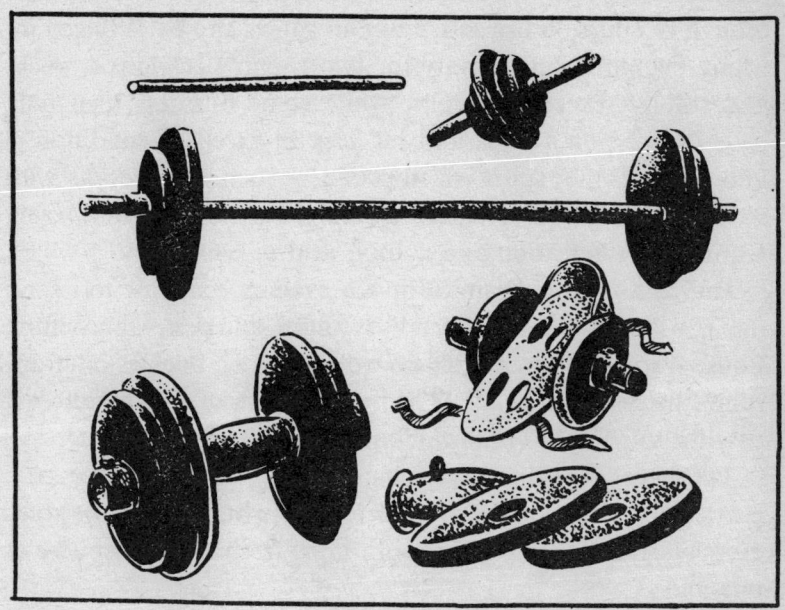

What a weight-training or body building set looks like: a steel rod, swingbell or centrally loaded dumbell, barbell, iron boots, a heavy dumbell, a dumbell sleeve and iron discs.

'outgrow' his weights. I mention these as they are two basic exercises that appear in all schedules, whether for the beginner or advanced bodybuilder. They will be fully described later.

METHOD OF TRAINING

A weight-training workout can last anything from 15 to 20 minutes up to 3 hours for the specialist, but the ideal is around 1 to 1½ hours according to the length of rest periods between exercises. The older person takes slightly longer to recover between exercises than the younger one will.

Most people who use weights train three times a week. Of course those who are keener train perhaps four times, but three is enough for the average individual. If possible there should be a complete rest day from weight training between each session, though of course other activities and games can be indulged in. Many people find time only for two training sessions a week, and still get excellent results, while some business men only have one session a week and yet keep in excellent condition. I know of no other sport which produces such good results with so little training, though it is only fair to say that weight training requires concentration and a good deal of hard work!

The best time to train is in the evening, but not too soon (never within one hour) after a heavy meal, and preferably before. Loose warm clothing should be worn, with no buckles or straps round the waist, and a pair of light slippers or even barefeet if conditions permit. Training boots can come later.

The usual precautions against catching cold are necessary, particularly as there are short periods of sitting about between exercises. Try to keep your room in as fresh an atmosphere as possible.

Before commencing any type of weight-training exercise it is essential to loosen up the muscles thoroughly with some freestanding exercises for about five minutes and I suggest that you take some of the exercises given in the freestanding tables. Ensure that all the joints and limbs are thoroughly loose before commencing, for this will minimize the risk of strain or stiffness.

THE SET SYSTEM

This is the most widely used of the modern methods of weight training to-day. There are of course other methods designed for the bodybuilding specialist, but even for him, the Set System is the most strongly advocated. The Set System is one I advocate not only for improving health and physique but also as an aid to other sports.

Briefly this system means that you do not do each exercise for so many repetitions, but you do several sets of repetitions for each exercise with a little breather between each set. The idea of this is to concentrate on one particular muscle area at a time, before proceeding to another one. By so doing the blood flow to any particular part is increased, and therefore not only strengthens but helps to enlarge and strengthen the muscles in that area.

To explain further, suppose you were doing an exercise for the upper arms three sets of 8 repetitions, (i.e. 24 times in all) we mean that you do a set of 8 repetitions, have a short breather, and then do 8 more, until you have completed three sets. Incidentally for the beginner 8—12 repetitions is the most common number to do, and three sets the most often used number of sets. You may have seen it written in technical magazines like this 3×8; it means that you do three sets of 8 repetitions.

Of course in some exercises it is practicable to do more, or less, than three sets, and with a complete beginner very often one set of any exercise is enough.

The commencing poundage to be used must be worked out by yourself. It is most important for the beginner to make sure that the exercise is done CORRECTLY AND WITH A FULL RANGE OF MOVEMENT, rather than struggling to use a heavier weight a smaller number of times. The one danger of this form of training, is that the beginner always wants to see how *much* he can lift. This practice is definitely not to be recommended. Remember it is much more important to do an exercise correctly for 8 repetitions, than to struggle to add more weight and do it once or twice.

Weight should only be increased when the requisite number of repetitions becomes *easy*. Sometimes this may not be for weeks, sometimes progress will be rapid.

Training with Weights at Home

Sometimes it is a good thing when planning your training, to add just a little weight (say 2½ lb.) for each set of an exercise, and so make each set a bit harder.

Now that I have given you some idea of the type of equipment for home training, the poundages, the method, you can turn to Chapter Eleven for an explanation of the best exercises, and then you will learn how to compile a training schedule for yourself. I will also give you a brief idea of the starting poundages to try, but do remember that this must depend on what weights you have, your age, and natural potentiality. If you cannot use the weight I recommend, or want to use more, it is up to you. This is just a guide for you to 'feel' the exercise.

There are one or two very valuable exercises that are difficult to do on your own, because of getting the heavier weight used into position by yourself. This indicates one of the advantages of having a training partner, or training at a club where they usually have stands or racks, etc., from which to take the weights and so make your training pleasanter and easier.

CHAPTER ELEVEN

A Vast Choice of Exercises for You

BARBELL—UPPER BODY

1. The Clean
2. Press with Barbell
3. Press Behind Neck
4. Straight Arm Pullover
5. Bent Arm Pullover
6. Bench Press
7. Upright Rowing
8. Bent over Rowing
9. 'Good Morning' Exercise
10. Dead Lift

BARBELL EXERCISES—ARMS

11. The Curl and Variations
12. Reverse Curl
13. Standing Triceps Stretch
14. Triceps Stretch Lying
15. Triceps Extension from the Hang

BARBELL EXERCISES—LEGS

16. The Squat
17. Squat with Weight at Clean

18. The Straddle Lift
19. The Hack Lift
20. Heels Raise with Barbell
21. Seated Heels Raise

BARBELL EXERCISES—ABDOMINAL

22. Sit Ups with Barbell

DUMBELL EXERCISES—UPPER BODY

23. Alternate Dumbell Press
24. Two Hands Dumbell Press
25. Dumbell Bench Press
26. Two Hand Dumbell Bench Press
27. Flying Exercise
28. Lateral Raise Sideways and Upwards
29. Alternate Forward and Upward Swings with Dumbells
30. One Hand Swing
31. Single Arm Rowing

DUMBELL EXERCISES—ARMS

32. Two Hands Dumbell Curls or Alternate Dumbell Curls
33. Single Arm Seated Dumbell Curl
34. Bent Over Single Arm Inward Curl
35. Lying Curl with Dumbells
36. Single Arm Triceps Stretch
37. Two Hands Single Dumbell Triceps Stretch
38. Single Arm Triceps Extension

LEG WORK WITH DUMBELLS

39. The Squat with Dumbells and Calf Raises
40. Single Leg Squat with Dumbell

LATERAL

41. Sidebends with Dumbells Single and (42) Double

SWINGBELL EXERCISES

43. Press with Swingbell
44. Press Behind Neck with Swingbell
45. Straight Arm Pullover with Swingbell
46. Bent Arm Pullover with Swingbell
47. Two Hands Swing with Swingbell
48. Forward and Upward Swing with Swingbell
49. Curl with Swingbell and Variations
50. Triceps Stretch with Swingbell
51. French Press with Swingbell
52. Sidebends with Swingbell

HOW TO PERFORM THE LISTED EXERCISES CORRECTLY

BARBELL EXERCISES

The first and most important thing to learn is how to pick the bar from the floor to the shoulders correctly, as this is the commencing position of many of the standing exercises. Taking the weight, i.e. the bar with discs at either end, from the floor to the shoulders is called the 'CLEAN'. The descriptive wording is 'CLEANING THE WEIGHT TO THE SHOULDERS'.

1. The Clean

Stand short astride, feet about 15 inches apart, insteps against the bar, feet underneath, and toes pointing to the front. Bend the knees and keeping the back quite flat, head and chest well up, grasp the weight with the thumbs round the bar KNUCKLES UPPERMOST. The width of the hands depends on the exercise you are doing, but for most it is slightly wider than shoulder width apart. In the initial position with the knees bent the arms are kept straight. Sink well back on the heels ensuring that they never leave the floor, and with a vigorous pull of the arms, straighten the legs and pull the bar upwards as high as possible towards the chest. When the bar is as high as it will go twist the wrists quickly and the bar should be in the 'clean' position high up across the shoulders and in line with the Adam's apple. Elbows must be kept well up, and the weight mostly on the ball part of the thumbs. SPEED IS ESSENTIAL in this movement which must be continuous, and the back and legs must bear the brunt of the work. For a complete beginner, I suggest that you practise cleaning and lowering the weight several times as an exercise. It is a very good back and leg strengthener, and also teaches you the balance necessary for the more advanced exercises.

2. Press with Barbell

From the clean position, already described, press the barbell to arms' length and lower it, making sure that each movement is complete, but that there is no long pause between repetitions. Keep the bar as near to the face as possible, and try not to lean back when pressing. Contract the thighs as the press is made, and also contract the buttocks, and pull your 'tail' in. Ensure that when you are at arms' length, that a final stretch is given to the shoulders before lowering the weight. Breathe in just as the press is made, and out as the weight is lowered. This is a great exercise for the back, deltoids, triceps, and chest generally. Suggest 30 lb. as a trial. You may find this very easy, for some fairly strong men have pressed as much as 100 lb. at their first attempt.

3. Press Behind Neck

From the clean to the shoulders position the weight is lifted over the head and lowered to rest on the back of the neck. A slightly wider grip is recommended. At the end of each press to arms' length ensure that the weight returns to touch the top of the spine at each repetition. This is a stronger exercise than the press, and is especially good for the upper back and triceps. The

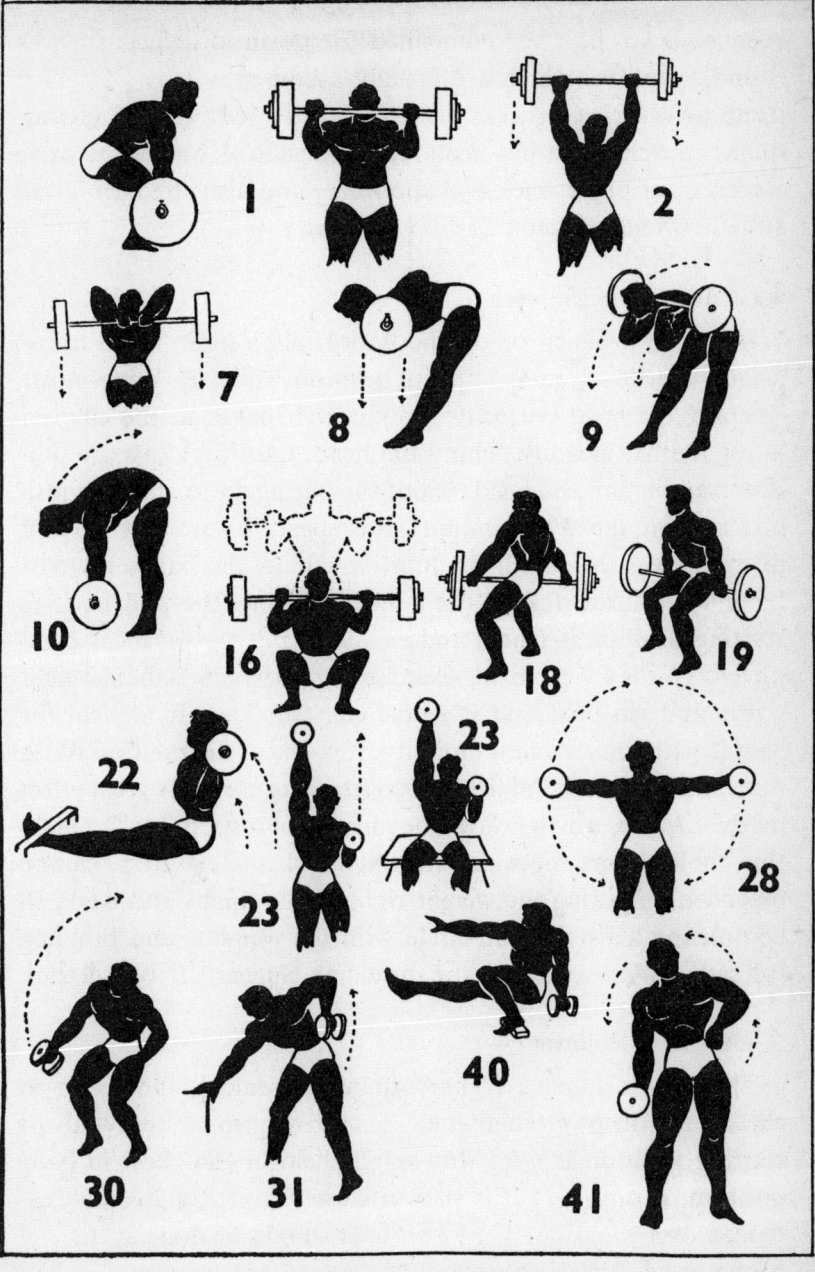

exercise is strongly recommended for postural defects such as round shoulders which are usually accompanied by shortened pectoral muscles. It also has a marked effect on the erector spinae muscles, and has been recommended as one of the basic exercises for upper back and shoulders and arm strength for all athletic events. Suggest 25 lb. as a trial.

4. Straight Arm Pullover

Lying on a bench or on the floor, hold a light bar at arms' length overhead, in overgrasp position knuckles uppermost. Keeping the arms perfectly straight and locked at the elbows, lower the bar steadily behind the head, until the arms are out-stretched behind the head. Raise the bar again to starting position keeping the arms straight, and repeat. Ensure that the hips do not leave the bench or floor. Inhale as the bar is lowered behind the head, take a deep breath just as the pull back to starting position is made, and exhale as the movement is completed. This is a very strong exercise for the whole of the shoulder girdle and rib box, and is a fine chest builder. It is ideal for people with limited chest mobility. It is one of the basic exercises recommended for athletics and sports, because of its great effect on the rib box, which houses the muscles of respiration. It makes the whole thorax more mobile and supple. The exercise can be extended by taking the weight right to the thighs and back, so completing a whole semi-circle with the weights, and bringing full range of movement to the shoulders. Suggest 15 lb. as a trial.

5. Bent Arm Pullover

This is best done as a 'short range' movement, and is a great chest and triceps strengthener. A narrow grip is used, and the starting position is with the weight held at the chest in lying position. From there it is passed closely over the face and extended over the edge of the bench. It should be done at the end of the bench for this purpose.

The weight is brought back to the starting position in a short range movement, breathing in as the weight is carried behind the head, out as it is brought back. Ensure that the hips remain on the bench or floor. It is better done on a bench so that the arms are carried well back and down with elbows bent. Suggest 30 lb. as a trial.

6. Bench Press

This exercise can be done on the floor, but is better done on a bench so that full play is given to the arms and chest, and movement is not restricted.

Lie on a bench or form, or a raised base with the shoulders firmly on it. Take a bar to arms' length, with a fairly wide grip. Lower the bar to the chest, and then press it overhead to arms' length, ensuring that it is kept fairly high up the chest, and not allowed to come too far towards the abdomen when it is lowered. Take a deep breath as you lower the bar to the chest, and breathe out as the press to arms' length is completed. This is a great exercise for the whole of the chest, pectorals, triceps, and some of the back muscles. It is one of the recommended basic exercises for all athletic events and sports. It is perfectly safe, and there is no fear of any injury. Suggest 50 lb. as a trial.

Note.—In all the exercises lying on a bench, it is better that the feet are kept firmly on the floor rather than on the bench, so that better balance can be maintained.

7. Upright Rowing

Stand short astride with the bar at the 'hang position' (i.e. hanging at arms' length) in front of the thighs, hands about 6 inches apart, knuckles to front. With a strong pull, bend the elbows, and keeping the bar as near to the body as possible, pull it up as high as possible in line with the neck, raising the elbows high. Lower to arms' length and repeat. Inhale as the weight is raised, exhale as it is lowered.

This is a great exercise for the deltoids, pectorals and chest generally. Suggest 25 lb. for a trial.

8. Bent Over Rowing

With the bar at the hang position, legs astride, bend forward until the body is at right angles to the legs. Keeping the back flat and staying in the forward position with the arms hanging in front, pull the bar up to the lower chest. A fairly wide grip is advocated for this exercise. Breathe deeply when pull is made, exhale as the weight is lowered. You can rest your forehead on a bench or table to help with this exercise. It is an excellent one for the back muscles, particularly the latissimus dorsi muscles, the trapezius, and triceps.

9. Good Morning Exercise

Stand astride with a barbell held behind the neck across the shoulders. From this position, bend the trunk forward, keeping the head well up, so that the bar does not slip forward. Try and bend at least to right angles with the legs. Return to upright and repeat. Inhale as you come up, exhale as you lower the trunk. This is a great lower back exercise, and is particularly good for posture as it stretches the hamstrings, the long tendons of the legs. Suggest 20 lb. for a trial.

10. Dead Lift

Stand short astride or feet together, feet under the bar toes to front. Keeping the back straight, bend the knees and grasp the bar with one hand overgrasp and one hand undergrasp, arms shoulder width apart. Using the back and leg muscles, straighten the legs, lifting the bar to the hang position. Brace the shoulders well back and lift the chest. This is a great all-round strengthening exercise, and for people who have had experience of weight training, can be done with straight legs. It strengthens the whole of the back, trapezius and triceps. It may not be suitable for home training, unless you have plenty of weights, as even a beginner would start around 100 lb. for this exercise.

ARM EXERCISES WITH BARBELL

Many of the exercises already described have a marked effect on the arms, mostly triceps and forearms, particularly exercises like the Press behind Neck, Bench Press, etc. But I now detail a few special exercises which have particular effect on the arms.

11. The Curl

This exercise has many variations, and in some form should appear in every weight training schedule. Many of the other exercises naturally affect the arm, but the curl has a very direct effect on the upper arm. The usual way of doing it is as follows: Stand short astride or feet together, hold a barbell at the hang position, arms shoulder width apart, palms to the front. Without any body or upper arm movement bend the elbows and 'curl' the bar upwards to the shoulders. Then lift the elbows well up. Inhale as the curl is made, exhale as the bar is lowered. When the curl is made a quick contraction takes place of the upper arm muscles. This exercise can be done wide or narrow grip, in slightly BENT FORWARD POSITION, SEATED or STANDING. All have their merits and work the upper arm muscles from varying angles. I suggest about 30 lb. for a trial.

12. Reverse Curl

This is the same as the curl, but with the knuckles to front. The bar is not taken so high as the curl, and the effect is mostly on the forearms and wrists. Twenty pounds for a trial.

13. Standing Triceps Stretch

Stand astride, and using a narrow grip, take the bar to over-head by pressing it, and grip as for press. From the arms extended position, lower the bar behind the head merely by dropping the forearms behind the head. The upper arm remains as still as possible With a contraction of the triceps muscles, stretch arms by straightening the elbows, until the bar is at its starting position. This exercise can also be done seated. Try 20 lb. for a start.

14. Triceps Stretch Lying

This exercise can be done at the end of a bench, in lying position. Hold a bar with narrow grip at arms' length overhead, keeping the upper arm straight drop the bar behind the head by bending the forearms backwards. Twenty pounds for a start.

15. Triceps Extension from the Hang

Stand astride hold a barbell shoulder width apart across the buttocks palms to front. Without any body movement and keeping the arms straight, take the bar further backwards from the shoulder and return. Feel the pull on the triceps muscles. Fifteen pounds for a start.

Note—MANY OF THESE EXERCISES LIKE THE PRESS, PRESS BEHIND NECK, ETC., CAN BE DONE STANDING OR SEATED FOR PROGRESSION.

LEG EXERCISES—THIGHS

16. The Squat

Like the Bench Press and Curl, this great exercise should, in some form, be in every schedule. It is not only a great leg and stamina builder, but because of its effect on the respiratory system it is also a great chest and body weight builder. It is one of the basic exercises for athletic events and sports.

Stand feet short astride, toes to front. With a barbell supported across the shoulders behind the neck, bend the knees and sink into a knees bend position. Immediately return to the upright. Inhale deeply just prior to the knees bend, and exhale as you come to the upright. Fill the lungs a couple of times before each repetition. The *back must be kept flat*. This is very important, on no account must the back be allowed to sag. If you are not too supple, do not squat too deeply, only until the thighs are slightly below parallel with the ground is sufficient. The heels must remain on the ground all the time. If you have difficulty in keeping the heels on the ground, raise them on a block of wood. I suggest 50 lb. for a trial.

17. Squat with Weight at Clean

The squat exercise can also be done with the weight held with a narrow grip at the front of the chest, in which case you will need a block under the heels. It throws more work on the front of the thighs and therefore strengthens them. Try 40 lb. for a start.

18. The Straddle Lift

Stand with one leg either side of a barbell, feet about 15 inches apart. Grasp the bar with one hand in front of the thighs and one to the rear, the barbell being fore and aft. Bend the knees and keeping the back flat, lift the bar from the floor by straightening the legs and using the back muscles. Try this with 60 lb. for a start.

19. Hack Lift

Stand short astride in FRONT of a barbell. Bend the knees and keeping the back flat, and with a slight forward incline of the body, grasp the bar knuckles to front or back as preferred. Using the back and legs, lift the bar off the floor and resume the upright position, and repeat. Inhale on lift, exhale on lower. Try with about 80 lb. for a start.

CALF EXERCISES

For many of the best exercises for calves no apparatus is

required for such movements as running, skipping, jumping, etc. on the toes. Even heels raising with toes on a block of wood is effective. However, more concentrated muscle work is possible when weights provide the resistance. Here are two special exercises.

20. Heels Raise with Barbell

Stand short astride toes to the front with a barbell supported on the shoulders. From this position raise on the toes as high as possible, hold position a second or so if possible, and lower, and repeat. Suggest about 50 lb. as a trial.

21. Seated Heels Raise

Sit on a chair or stool with a loaded barbell resting on a towel across the knees, with toes on a block of wood. Raise the heels as high as possible, and lower.

This is a very effective exercise for developing stubborn çalf muscles which have failed to respond to other work.

22. Sit Ups with Barbell

This is an advanced abdominal exercise, but I will include it as it can be used for home training. With the bar held behind the neck or at the chest and in lying position, and the FEET FIXED under another object, sit up with the weight until the body is upright, then resume the lying position. Inhale prior to the sit up, exhale as you come up. Beginners will find this difficult at first and may have to be content to use only the bar without weights.

*   *   *

These are but a few of the barbell exercises that can be done at home by a beginner with a light set. There are of course many more and I will add some more advanced exercises in a later chapter on training in the gym or at a club.

A Vast Choice of Exercises for You

I will give you a trial schedule taken from these exercises, so that you can see for yourselves what a workout would look like. I suggest that this is suitable for a complete beginner, and the number of sets of each exercise recommended can be increased after a dozen or so actual training sessions. You do each exercise for one or more SETS, each set being of so many repetitions.

FOR A COMPLETE BEGINNER

General loosening up with freestanding exercises. Then take these exercises in any order preferred, but I recommend this sequence:

SQUAT WITH BARBELL (Ex. 16). Two sets of 8—10 repetitions
PULLOVER ON BENCH (Ex. 4). Two sets of 8—10 repetitions
PRESS BEHIND NECK (Ex. 3). Two sets of 8 repetitions
CURL (Ex. 11). Three sets of 8 repetitions
BENCH PRESS (Ex. 6). Three sets of 8 repetitions
BENT OVER ROWING (Ex. 8). Two sets of 8 repetitions.
CALF RAISES (Freestanding). ABDOMINAL EXERCISES. Three sets taken from Freestanding schedules.

Note.—At first you may not be able to do the required number of repetitions in each set, but these are what you want to aim for. Do what you can at first until you are used to the routine.

The workout should be done comfortably in an hour, allowing for short rests between each set `and each exercise. I suggest three workouts a week as ideal to allow tissues to be replaced and muscles to grow. Of course other activities can be taken on other days, but try not to indulge in pastimes which make big demands on your energy.

Most of the barbell exercises described can also be done with dumbells, or a CENTRALLY LOADED DUMBELL ROD, which is known as a SWINGBELL and which is excellent for many exercises such as the CURL, PULLOVER, TRICEPS STRETCH, ETC.

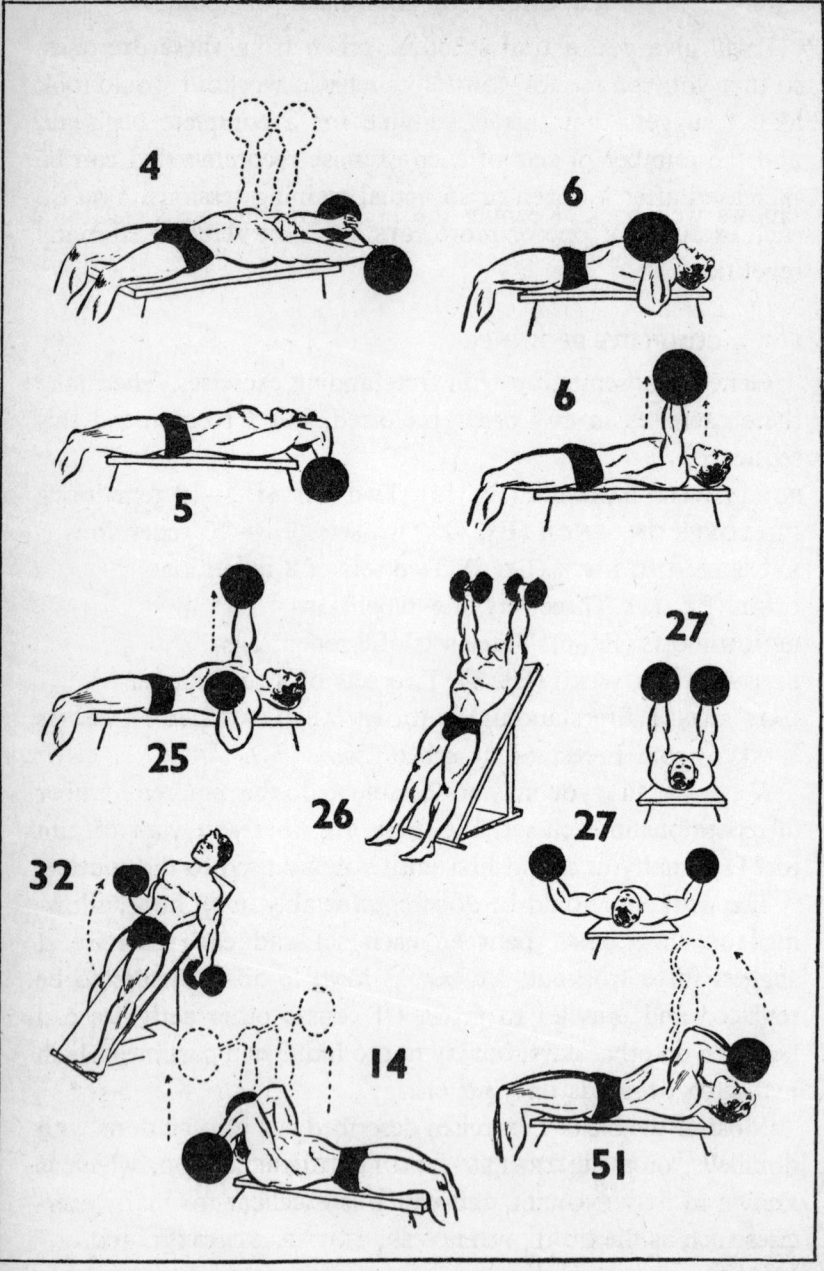

DUMBELL EXERCISES—UPPER BODY

23. Alternate Dumbell Press

Stand feet together or short astride. Using legs and back as for the CLEAN (Ex. 1) lift a pair of dumbells to the shoulders, elbows well back. Keeping the body straight, press the right dumbell overhead and lower to shoulder, simultaneously pressing the left dumbell overhead. To maintain balance keep the dumbells as near to the head as possible when pressing. Breathe freely. This is an upper back, chest and deltoid exercise. Suggest 15 lb. each dumbell for a trial.

24. Two Hands Dumbell Press

This is the same exercise as above, but more advanced, and of course both dumbells are pressed together instead of alternately. Poundage as above.

25. Dumbell Bench Press Alternate

As in Exercise 6 with barbell. Take a pair of dumbells to the shoulders whilst lying down. Press them alternately above the head. Breathe freely. Suggest 20 lb. each dumbell for a trial.

26. Two Hands Dumbell Bench Press

The same exercise as above, but press overhead with both dumbells simultaneously. The exercise is more effective if the wrists are turned as the dumbells are lowered to the chest, so that the dumbells are turned from parallel overhead to in line at the chest. Both these are excellent chest and triceps exercises. Poundage as above. Breathing as for Exercise 6.

27. Flying Exercise

From the Bench Press position lower the arms, slightly bent outwards. Return to straight arms. Refer illustration 27, previous page. It is a fairly advanced exercise more for the pectoral muscles. Suggest 10 lb. each dumbell.

28. Lateral Raise Sideways and Upwards

Stand astride with a dumbell in each hand, arms at the hang position. Raise the dumbells, keeping the arms straight and body erect, until they are at right angles to the body. Then turn the wrists outwards so that the palms of the hands are upwards and carry the movement until the dumbells are above the head. Lower in the same way, making the upward and downward movements continuous with a turn of the wrists. This is a fine shoulder, deltoid and latissimus movement. Try it with 8 lb. on each dumbell for a start.

29. Alternate Forward and Upward Swings with Dumbells

Stand short astride with a dumbell held in each hand across the thighs, knuckles to front, dumbells held longwise. Alternate swing forward and upward with shoulder press. Ensure that there is no body movement. This is a fine shoulder and pectoral movement. Try it with 8 lb. each dumbell as a start.

30. One Hand Swing

Stand astride, bend over and grasp a dumbell placed between the feet. Bend the knees, keep the back flat, and keeping the lifting arm straight, straighten the legs and swing the dumbell overhead to arms' length. Allow the dumbell to swing back to starting position between the legs and repeat. Be careful to maintain balance. A strong shoulder and back exercise. Try with a 10 lb. dumbell. Later on when you handle heavier weights you will need to move the feet, taking one foot forward and the other back in the form of a lunge as the weight goes to arms' length overhead.

31. Single Arm Rowing

Holding a dumbell in one hand, lean forward at the waist. Place the free hand on a bench or chair for support. Vigorously pull the bell up to the shoulder as high as possible, keeping the trunk in the bent over position. Do not alter the position of the trunk, and lift the dumbell as high as possible in a rowing motion. This is a fine latissimus dorsi exercise. Try it with a 10 lb. dumbell.

ARMS

The Curl, Bent over Curl, Seated or Standing Curl (Ex. 11) in the Barbell series, can be done with a SWINGBELL or centrally loaded dumbell as already stated. The SEATED SWINGBELL CURL is particularly good. The swingbell is held at the hang position between the legs, and is curled by bending the elbows. The body remains with a slight lean forward.

32. Two Hands Dumbell Curls or Alternate Dumbell Curls

Stand astride with the arms at the hang position holding a dumbell in each hand. Fully flex the elbows and curl each dumbell alternately to the shoulder, or as a more advanced exercise, both dumbells can be curled together. This exercise can also be done seated, or in the bent over position, which provides even stronger work. There should be no body movement when the exercises are done in the standing position. For a trial use two 10 lb. dumbells. These, like the Barbell curls, are fine exercises for the upper arm.

In this exercise the dumbells should be kept in line from the starting position palms outward, and not parallel.

33. Single Arm Seated Dumbell Curl

Seated on a stool or bench, hold a dumbell between the knees with the arm extended. Flex the elbow and curl the dumbell to the shoulder. The trunk should be slightly inclined forward to produce a maximum contraction of the elbow flexors. A certain amount of support is possible by having the back of the elbow

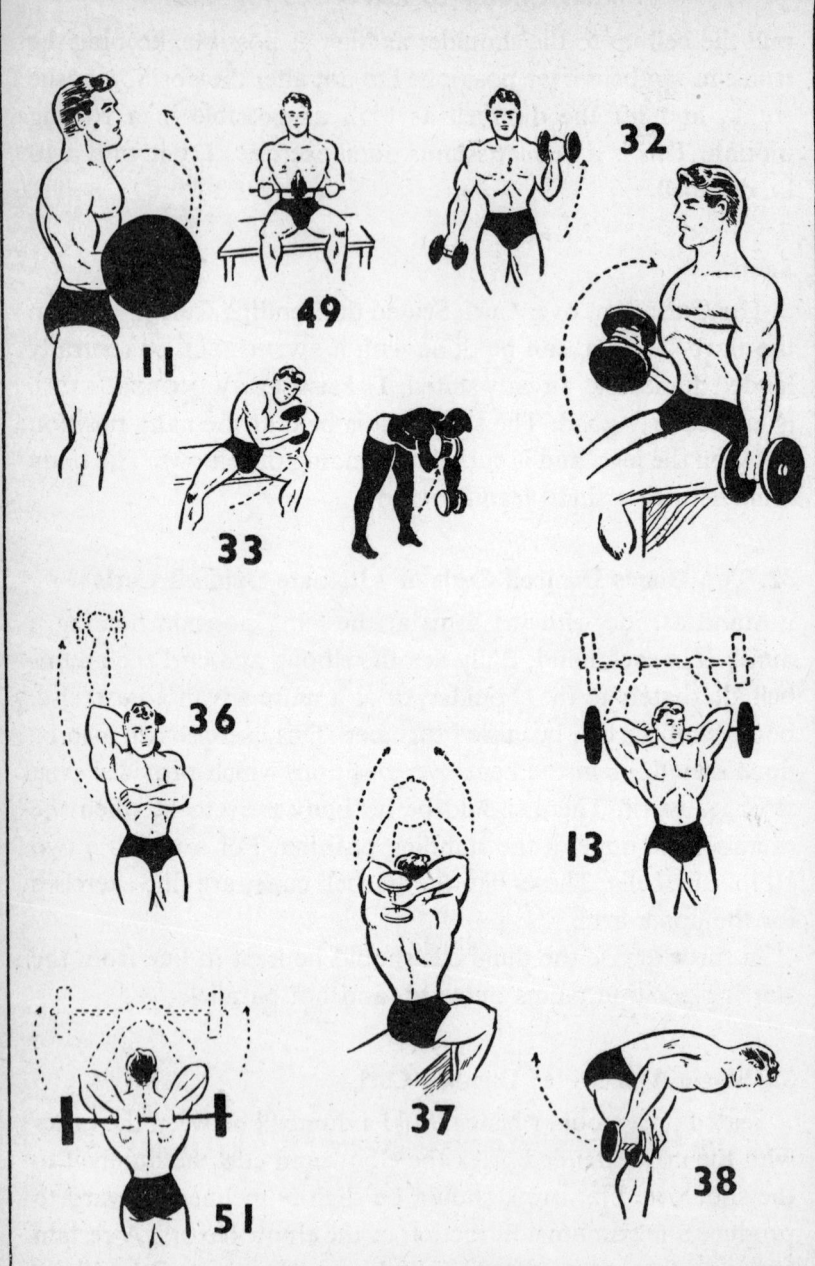

against the inside of the leg. Try with a 10 lb. dumbell. Also a
fine upper arm exercise.

34. Bent Over Single Arm Inward Curl

Bend the trunk forward, and holding a dumbell at the hang
position, with the other hand on a chair or stool for support,
curl the dumbell inwards towards the chest, instead of upwards
by flexing the elbow. This exercise produces a different type of
contraction of the biceps muscles, and is very much harder than
the ordinary curl. Try with 10 lb. as a start.

35. Lying Curl with Dumbells

Lying on a bench holding a dumbell in each hand with arms
in the hang position at either side of the bench, and palms to the
front so that dumbells are in line, curl the dumbells to the
shoulders. This is an advanced exercise, but I will include it
for home training. Try with 8 lb. on each dumbell.

36. Single Arm Triceps Stretch

Using a light dumbell, hold it at arms' length above the head.
Lower the dumbell backwards behind the head, by bending the
elbow until the dumbell touches the back of the neck. Then
keeping the upper arm straight, and by contracting the triceps
muscles straighten the forearm until the dumbell returns to
starting position. Keep the dumbell as near to the head as
possible all the time. The free arm is laid across the upper chest
for support on the side that is being exercised. Inhale at commencing position, exhale as movement is completed. This is a
very strong triceps exercise. Try with a 5 lb. dumbell for a start.

37. Two Hands Single Dumbell Triceps Stretch

Holding a single dumbell with both hands over each other
round the centre, press the dumbell overhead until arms are
quite straight, then lower the dumbell behind the back of the

head by bending the forearms backwards, until the dumbell touches the back of the shoulders. Keeping the upper arms fixed straighten the elbows by contracting the triceps muscles. This is a very good exercise for a beginner, and not so advanced as the one above. Try with a 10 lb. dumbell for a start.

38. Single Arm Triceps Extension

Stand astride with trunk bent forward at right angles. Holding a light dumbell at the hang position palm to front, carry the dumbell backwards without using the body. Action is from the arm and shoulder of arm holding the dumbell only. The free hand can be used for support. This exercise has a very strong triceps action. I suggest 8 lb. as a trial.

LEG WORK WITH DUMBELLS

39. Squat with Dumbells

Exercise 17 THE SQUAT with Barbell can be done also with dumbells, holding them either at the shoulders, or in the hang position.

Calf work can also be done holding the dumbells in the hang position and performing the heels raise. Or SINGLE LEG CALF RAISES can be done by holding one dumbell and using the free hand for support. The dumbell should be on the side that is being exercised, thus providing more resistance.

40. Single Leg Squat with Dumbell

Holding a dumbell in one hand and supporting yourself with the free hand on a chair or against a wall, perform a single leg squat holding the dumbell on the side which is being exercised. For more freedom of movement, this exercise can be done standing on a chair seat and supporting oneself on the back of the chair with the free hand. This is a very strong exercise, and should be practised without a dumbell at first, and then progress to a very light dumbell.

41. Sidebends with Single Dumbells

Stand feet together holding a dumbell in the right hand. Bend sideways from the waist as far as possible to the right, and return to the starting position. Concentrate on keeping the body straight, and let the neck and head move freely. Repeat on the left side. Try with a 10 lb. dumbell.

42. Sidebends with Dumbells

Stand astride with a dumbell in each hand. Trunk bend from side to side freely, with head and neck relaxed. Pull dumbell well up sideways on side opposite to the one bending. Don't sway forwards or backwards; keep the body moving in a sideways motion only. Try with a 5 lb. dumbell in each hand.

SWINGBELL

I have already mentioned the use of a SWINGBELL or centrally loaded dumbell rod, but for easy reference I will enumerate some of the exercises and give them a number;

43. Press with Swingbell

Done as Exercise 2 with barbell.

44. Press Behind Neck with Swingbell

Done as Exercise 3 with barbell.

45. Straight Arm Pullover with Swingbell

Done as Exercise 4 with barbell.

46. Bent Arm Pullover with Swingbell

Done as Exercise 5 with barbell.

47. Two Hands Swing with Swingbell

This is slightly different from any counterpart with dumbell or barbell. Grasp a swingbell in front of the thighs with both hands, standing well astride, bend forward until the swingbell is at the feet. From this position swing the bell overhead in one single movement, finishing with the arms straight, and return to starting position with bell at feet and repeat in rhythmic movements. Try with a swingbell weighing 10 lb. Keep arms straight all the time and maintain balance.

48. Forward and Upward Raise with Swingbell

This is the same as the exercise above, but the body is not bent forward, and the movement is taken from the standing position only.

49. Curl with Swingbell

This is taken as Exercise 11 with barbell and can be done STANDING, SEATED or IN BENT OVER POSITION. The seated curl with swingbell is strongly recommended for beginners. I suggest 30 lb. as a trial.

50. Triceps Stretch with Swingbell

This is done as Exercise 13 with barbell, and can be done STANDING, SEATED or LYING. I suggest 20 lb. for a trial.

51. French Press with Swingbell

This is a version of the Triceps Stretch, but done at the end of a bench, with the hands held in reverse position knuckles to front, as for curls. Lie on the end of a bench, the swingbell at arms length above the head. Lower the bell behind the head by bending the forearms backwards behind the head. By contracting the triceps, straighten the arms, trying to keep the upper arm still. Try with 20 lb. for a start.

52. Sidebends with Swingbell

Stand astride, arms above the head holding a swingbell.

Trunk bend from side to side. This is a very strong lateral exercise. I recommend 10 lb. for a trial.

Here then are some of the best known exercises for use with dumbells and SWINGBELL (which of course can be made up from a single dumbell rod and suitable disc weights). These exercises should give you vast scope for home training even if you only have a light dumbell set. Here is a simple schedule for a BEGINNER WITH DUMBELLS AND SWINGBELL only:

Warm up with freestanding exercises taken from the earlier schedules. Then take the following exercises in this order:

ALTERNATE DUMBELL PRESS (Ex. 23). Two sets of 8 repetitions each side.

PRESS ON BENCH WITH DUMBELLS (Ex. 26). Three sets of 8 repetitions.

SQUAT with dumbells held at the hang position, heels on block (Ex. 39). Three sets of 10 repetitions.

PULLOVER ON BENCH WITH SWINGBELL (Ex. 45 done as Ex. 4). Three sets of 8 repetitions.

SEATED SWINGBELL CURL (Ex. 49 done as Ex. 11 with barbell). Three sets of 8 repetitions.

DUMBELL TRICEPS STRETCH (Ex. 37). Three sets of 8 repetitions.

ABDOMINALS taken from freestanding exercises.

SIDEBENDS (Ex. 42) with dumbells one set to count of twenty-four.

CALF RAISES freestanding.

This should take about one hour with rests, etc., as for the barbell schedule.

Finally for those who have a combined Barbell and Dumbell set, here is a suggested schedule for you:

Warm up with freestanding exercise, then taken in any order preferred:

PRESS BEHIND NECK (Ex. 3). Two sets of 8 repetitions, increase to three sets later.

SQUAT (Ex. 16). Three sets of 10 repetitions.

CURL WITH BARBELL (Ex. 11). Three sets of 8 repetitions.

BENCH PRESS (Ex. 6). Three sets of 8 repetitions.

SINGLE ARM TRICEPS STRETCH (Ex. 36). Three sets of 8 repetitions each arm.

BENT OVER ROWING (Ex. 8). With barbell, three sets of 8 repetitions.

LATERAL RAISE WITH DUMBELLS (Ex. 28). Two sets of 8 repetitions.

ABDOMINALS from freestanding tables.

CALF work.

This is a simple schedule for beginners.

FIFTEEN-MINUTE SCHEDULE FOR A BUSINESS MAN

1. Warm up with Alternate Toe Touch 15 times.
   Stand astride trunk bend side to side 15 times.
   Skip with high knee raise, no rope.   2 mins.
2. Press with Barbell, 10 repetitions (Ex. 2).
3. Squat with Barbell, 12 repetitions (Ex. 16).
4. Good Morning Exercise, 12 repetitions (Ex. 9).
5. Upright Rowing, 12 repetitions (Ex. 7).
6. Bent Arm Pullover, 12 repetitions (Ex. 5).
7. Back lying legs raise to right angles 15 times.
8. Back lying knees raise to chest 15 times.
9. Deep Breathing-back lying, knees raise, feet on floor. 1 min.

I am confident that the whole of such a little schedule could be done comfortably in fifteen minutes and that every part of the body will have been exercised. I feel that many such little schedules can be compiled for the busy man or student from the very large selection of exercises at your disposal. These will keep you strong and healthy and ward off that middle-age spread.

CHAPTER TWELVE

Join a Health Studio or a Class

Training in a well-equipped bodybuilding gymnasium or studio has definite advantages over training at home, but the actual difference in the *method* of training is very little. The exercises are the same, but of course there are usually more pieces of apparatus, varying lengths of bars, dumbells, iron boots, etc., in fact so many appliances, that you may be a bit confused at first what you should use and what you should avoid. Many people who join a gym have a go at everything. They end by drifting from one piece of equipment to another, without any planned campaign of training, and without any ultimate goal. As a result they soon lose interest because they fail to achieve the results they have read so much about.

All the appliances have their use, but some are only really necessary for the specialist, or if a change of training is required. Interest must be maintained, monotony and staleness are things which must be avoided.

Training in a gym with others has very definite advantages. There is usually more room. You may find someone about your own standard to train with, or a couple of companions, and by comparison and results can make your training much more interesting.

In a gym you are able to handle more weight on your own in certain exercises such as the SQUAT (Ex. 16), and the BENCH PRESS (Ex. 6), because you can take the loaded barbells from stands or you can have the assistance of companions to lift the weights in place for you.

If you decide to join a bodybuilding club make up your mind from the start what you are aiming for. It may be to get fitter and stronger for some other sport, it may merely be to keep fit and get stronger for your daily job, or it may be to specialize in body-building and build yourself a physique of which to be proud. All these objects are slightly different, and your training plan should be selected accordingly.

TERMS THAT MAY PUZZLE

TYPE TRAINING

In Chapter Three we told you something about the varying types of physique, and how many people are naturally stocky, whilst others are naturally thin. A great deal has been written in the past about training to suit your type. This is a long and difficult subject, about which there is a great deal of difference of opinion. There are certain exercises like The Squat (Ex. 16), The Bench Press (Ex. 6), The Bent Over Rowing (Ex. 8), when done with heavy weights, that are considered to be 'bulk' pro-ducing exercises. Generally speaking, however, and for the majority, the guide is this: If you want to gain bulk (i.e. extra body weight) try and use heavy weights, with several sets of low repetitions (meaning about six repetitions to a set). If you want to build definition and cut down on your bulk, then train with lighter weights, and use several sets of high repetitions such as 12—15 each set.

In modern bodybuilding, there are many ways and many opinions of training. Some people advise only two or three basic exercises using many sets of low repetitions on the exer-cises. Others will tell you to do a large variety of exercises up to twelve or fifteen, so that you are using the muscles from every angle in a variety of movements. Interest in bodybuilding grows every year; there are new appliances, there are new methods, there are sweeping claims that this form or that form of training produces astonishing results. You cannot be expected to try all these, you will only get confused and bewildered. What may suit one person and his type, may be hopeless for you. There are the factors of your physical make-up, bone lengths, leverage, etc., to be considered. Some people have long legs while others have short ones. Some have long thighs and short lower legs, others short thighs and long lower legs and so on. All these factors may or may not retard your progress. In this book I have set out to deal with the AVERAGE individual, and I have recommended a sane and straightforward method of training. I have told you that the SET SYSTEM is the one I advocate, and for the majority, this will be all they need, with varying sets and varying repetitions according to their requirements. However, in case you already have some experience in bodybuilding and read the various P.C. journals and wondered what some of the terms mean, I will explain a few:

CHEATING METHODS

This is a favourite phrase of a training plan often used by advanced bodybuilders, the principle being to handle more weight and so get added bulk and strength, whether the exercise is done correctly or not. In other words if you are doing a CURL (Ex. 11) you try and *force* the weights up even if you have to use a body swing to do so, the theory being that the upper arm still gets the bigger percentage of the work, and with more weight the muscles work harder against the extra resistance.

FLUSHING

This is a method of doing very rapid repetitions of certain exercises with light weights, in order to produce a quick flow of blood to the muscles. The exercise is done very rapidly and therefore style is sacrificed to speed. It has its merits in certain advanced bodybuilding techniques. The theory is that the extra blood flushed to the muscles produces greater repair to the broken-down tissues.

CRAMPING OR CONCENTRATION MOVEMENTS

This is a method of doing short range movements with heavy weights to produce maximum 'pumping up' of the muscle. Short range Bent Arm Pullovers (Ex. 8) for instance. Short range Curls (Ex. 11), without extending the arms to full length. Half-range Press Behind Neck (Ex. 3). These movements may produce fine results and quick results, but because a muscle is not used through its full range of movement it gets shortened in time, restricting the full action of the joint over which the muscle works. This form of training over a period gives rise to many minor joint and muscular troubles. It is all right in its place, but should never be practised regularly for any length of time.

SUPER SETS

This is quite a good method of training for special cases. You do two exercises consecutively instead of one until it is finished. In other words you do an exercise like Curl (Ex. 11) for the upper arm, then follow with one for the Triceps like Dips between bars. In other words you are doing a compensatory exercise. And this is done until you complete so many sets of each exercise. Many people like to follow a set of Squats (Ex. 16), with a set of Straight Arm Pullovers (Ex. 4), as a compensatory exercise to restore the breathing to normal. They will do these alternately until the requisite number of sets of each exercise are done. It is a good idea for exercises that can be matched up like this.

BARBELL LENGTHS

The varying length of steel bars in a gym may puzzle you. If you are a beginner, it is best to use a medium length bar for most of the exercises, as they are easier to balance, with perhaps a longer bar for Squats. The shorter the bar, the heavier the weights will *seem* to you. Put 100 lb. on a long bar and press it overhead, and then 100 lb. on a short bar, and you will be amazed at the difference, which is only, actually, in the springiness of the bar. The weight, of course, is slightly more in a longer bar.

For arm and shoulder work short bars, or dumbells, are recommended; for bench pressing, squats, etc. the longer bar. Pullovers; Bent Arm Pullovers, etc., that need more control are better done with a short bar or swingbell.

If you have plenty of equipment at your disposal try to include in your workout a percentage of barbell exercises, and a percentage of dumbell exercises. Always include a couple of overhead exercises such as Press, Press behind neck, Dumbell presses, etc. Far too many people do too many lying down exercises, and therefore neglect the Erector Spinae muscles. A well-balanced workout should comprise about ten exercises to include abdominals. I suggest two should be done above the head, barbell, dumbells, pulley, etc., two good arm exercises, three general chest exercises, and the three trunk and abdominal exercises. The Squat (Ex. 16), and the Bench Press (Ex. 6) should come in every schedule in some form. The Bench Press can be done on a flat or inclined bench, declined, etc., with barbell or dumbells. There should always be some form of Curl (Ex. 11) in one of the many different ways it can be performed. There should always be one good triceps exercise such as Press Behind Neck (Ex. 3) or one of the many suggested triceps exercises. There should always be one or two strength exercises like the Press (Ex. 2), or Press Behind Neck (Ex. 3), also a good exercise like Dead Lift (Ex. 10).

With the use of more weight, many exercises suggested in the last chapter can be done in the gym. Dead Lifts (Ex. 10), are difficult to do unless one has sufficient weight.

There are one or two exercises I have not included in the previous chapter, but we have explained that they are variations of these but done on Inclined or Declined benches. Otherwise the exercises are exactly the same.

There are one or two exercises I deliberately omitted in the previous chapter because to do them at home is not so easy as they are inclined to be noisy, and also because the movement needs a good deal of technique.

THE SNATCH

In this exercise, a highly technical one, the weight is carried overhead from the floor in a single sharp movement. The bar is grasped with a wide grip, feet short astride, arms straight, knees bent, back flat. The weight is then pulled vigorously upwards as high as possible and then by moving the feet fore and aft the weight is carried over head. Then the upright position is regained. This exercise needs a good deal of tuition, and is a great one for building speed and co-ordination. I would recommend it in the Athletic schedules but feel that it is a bit advanced to be understood without individual instruction. It is also one of the three Olympic lifts.

Assuming that you have a fully equipped gym at your disposal, I will suggest three or four schedules for you:

A BEGINNER

General warm up with freestanding exercises. Followed by one Set of light Presses (Ex. 2) 10 quick, but complete, repetitions. Taken in any order:

SQUAT (Ex. 16). Three sets of 10 repetitions.

BENCH PRESS (Ex. 6). Three sets of 8 repetitions.

PRESS BEHIND NECK (Ex. 3). Three sets of 8 repetitions.

SINGLE ARM SEATED CURL (Ex. 33). Two sets of 8 repetitions each arm.

SEATED SWINGBELL CURL (Ex. 49). Two sets of 8 repetitions.

PULLEY TO BACK OF NECK (Ex. 2) Pulley Page 84. Three sets of 8 repetitions.

DIPS BETWEEN PARALLEL BARS. Three sets of 8 repetitions.
ABDOMINAL EXERCISES taken from freestanding schedules.
SIDEBENDS.
CALF RAISES.

There you have a complete training session which gives a thorough work-out to the whole body.

SUGGESTED INTERMEDIATE SCHEDULE

Warm up with freestanding exercises as before.

Light repetition Presses Behind Neck (Ex. 3), one set of 10 repetitions.

ALTERNATE DUMBELL PRESS (Ex. 23). Three sets of 8 repetitions.

UPRIGHT ROWING (Ex. 7). Three sets of 8 repetitions.

SQUAT (Ex. 16). Three sets of 10 repetitions adding 10 lb. for each set.

BENCH PRESS (Ex. 6). Three sets of 10 repetitions adding 10 lb. each set.

ALTERNATE DUMBELL CURL (Ex. 32). Two sets of 8 repetitions.

SINGLE ARM INWARD CURL (Ex. 34). Two sets of 8 repetitions.

FRENCH PRESS WITH SWINGBELL (Ex. 51). Three sets of 8 repetitions.

DEAD LIFTS (Ex. 10). Four sets of 3 repetitions adding 10 lb. each set.

SIT UPS WITH BARBELL (Ex. 22). Three sets of 10 repetitions.

BACK LYING LEGS RAISE TO TOUCH FLOOR BEHIND HEAD. Two sets of 15.

CALF RAISES ON CALF MACHINE OR HEEL RAISES WITH BARBELL

SIDEBENDS WITH DUMBELL (Ex. 41). One set of 30.

AN ADVANCED SCHEDULE

Warm up as before.

TWO HANDS DUMBELL PRESS (Ex. 24). Three sets of 6 repetitions.

FLYING EXERCISE DONE ON INCLINED BENCH (Ex. 27). Three sets of 8 repetitions.

HEAVY SQUATS (Ex. 16). Four sets of 6 repetitions.

STRADDLE LIFT (Ex. 18). One set of 8 repetitions.

DUMBELL BENCH PRESS ON INCLINED BENCH (Ex. 25). Four sets of 8 repetitions.

BARBELL CURL NARROW GRIP LEAN FORWARD (Ex. 11). Three sets of 8 repetitions.

SEATED TRICEPS STRETCH (Ex. 13). Three sets of 8 repetitions.

BENT OVER ROWING (Ex. 8). Three sets of 8 repetitions.

ABDOMINALS SELECTED FROM IRON BOOT WORK. Four sets.

CALF WORK WITH CALF MACHINE.

These are but three schedules to give you some idea of the form a workout should take. Later on, if you wish you can work alternately on dumbell work and barbell work. You may like at some time to work specially on some weak point such as your arms, in which case you select three or four good exercises for the biceps and triceps, and work on these. Specialization on individual parts is NOT advocated unless for a special purpose. The whole aim should be for ALL ROUND DEVELOPMENT, STRENGTH, and above all else—HEALTH.

CHAPTER THIRTEEN

Weights Give the Sportsman that Extra Lift

For a sprinter there is no substitute for sprinting. The same goes for footballers, cricketers, tennis players, swimmers, etc. There is no substitute for the actual practising of essential techniques. I do not want to offer you a substitute or a short cut or a secret. All I want to do is to point out that weight training will vastly improve your performance.

No matter what sport you suggest nearly all the top men and many of the women to-day, have strengthened up with weight training. It has become normal practice.

I am certain that in the last Olympic Games a huge percentage of all male competitors had at some time done weight training, and an ever increasing number of women too.

Australian Lew Hoad, the famous tennis player, used to work up to three hours a night with the weights. Lynn Davies, the Olympic long jumper and gold medallist, has used weights for several years. His exercises include stepping on and off a bench with a 300-lb. barbell on his shoulders. Famous golfer Gary Player of South Africa trains with weights to 'unwind' after the tension of major tournaments and in fact was once the owner of a health studio where he trained himself.

Colin Campbell, one of Britain's top 400-metre men has trained with weights at a London evening institute for several years, and I have had the privilege of being one of the instructors at the same place.

All American athletes usually go into the gym to strengthen up during their competitive careers, and even during the season.

The Australian Herb Elliott, unbeaten in the mile and 1,500 metres, sparked off a revolution in athletics a few years ago by including an astonishing amount of heavy weight training in his workouts after many had 'dabbled' for quite a number of years.

So did Peter Snell, the famous New Zealand double gold medallist.

The main reason for the slow catch-on was that officials and coaches failed to see that strength via weight training could be harnessed to speed and co-ordination, and it was also necessary to break down prejudice and overcome ignorance of modern weight training techniques. Athletes and sportsmen in turn could only listen to the advice of the officials and coaches to whom they turned for advice.

The biggest snag, of course, was that those who knew a great deal about weight training knew nothing about the sports involved or the techniques required, but over the years this is gradually righting itself. Coaches and officials are usually against some new-fangled methods, simply because they never used them in their day.

It all started in Britain as long ago as 1948 when the Olympic Games were held in London and it was found that already American, and some continental, athletes and sportsmen had 'discovered' weights. Yet, as a keen sportsman myself, I found that weights had assisted me in any sport I had participated in until the age of forty, even if in a modest way; and many of my colleagues used weights to advantage for sport forty years ago.

When weight training for sports did catch on the usual crowd of fakes jumped on the bandwaggon and touted their 'expert' knowledge around. This did not help one little bit.

Now, in the evolution of sports, and as sportsmen and athletes have ended their careers and become coaches or officials, they can, as participators, pass on their methods of training to the younger generation.

So now we can really see what a great help weight training has been to sportsmen and women in all spheres of sport.

It can help you, too; not by finding out what some famous sportsman did for his event and then copying him, hoping to be good, but by finding out what suits you and where your weakness lies. In this respect you must experiment just as you do with your other skills.

There is no real need for a special schedule for each particular event or sport. The basic exercises are suitable for *any* sport for gaining strength, speed and even co-ordination, and certainly confidence.

It used to be the practice for a weight trainer, when he was approached by a footballer, to think to himself: 'This man needs strong legs,' and so give him many different leg exercises when already the footballer, through his training and playing, was exercising the leg muscles more than any other of the muscle groups. This is a very common mistake. By all means strengthen up any weakness in the muscle-groups you use for your sport, but also include some work for the muscles that may get little work at all from your particular sport or event. In this way you will balance the whole physique, lessen the chances of injury and improve speed and strength.

For instance, there are few sports or events where a performer could not do with a strong mid-section and stronger shoulders and chest. Remember, the chest contains the vital organs such as the heart, lungs and all the internal organs. All need strengthening to stand the rigours of modern sports techniques.

I feel that apart from the normal type of limbering up that each athlete already does for his event, four or five basic exercises like some form of Press, Squats (Deep Knee Bends), Pullover at Arms' Length, Bench Presses, Good Morning Exercise and with perhaps some Dead Lifts, and plenty of Abdominal work, should be the basis of every schedule, whether for running, jumping or field events, as I am quite convinced that these exercises alone will produce strength, and stamina without reducing speed or co-ordination. As mentioned earlier, however, a lighter weight should be used than those used by purely bodybuilding enthusiasts, and the exercise must be done in strict style with FULL RANGE OF MOVEMENT. No particular poundage can be fixed, for this is for the individual athlete to decide according to his capabilities. I have, however, made some suggestions in the schedule, worked out from average data that I have.

The ideal number of repetitions for each exercise is recommended as 8—12, but these must be varied slightly according to the event. Each exercise should be repeated for THREE SETS—that means that the exercise is done for say 10 repetitions, then a short rest is taken, and the exercise is repeated again, until three sets have been completed.

THE PRESS

STANDING PRESS (Ex. 2, page 106). Lift the bar to the chest in the correct way described under 'The Clean', Ex. 1, page 105. Press the barbell overhead, ensuring that the shoulders are fully stretched and the arms locked but without raising the heels from the floor. Look straight in front of you and never at the bar, for this will throw you off balance.

Repeat fairly rapidly, breathing in fully just as you press the bar overhead and exhaling as you return the bar to the chest.

This is a fine exercise for shoulders and upper back.

Let me explain these exercises and examine their merits as far as athletes are concerned:

THE SQUAT OR KNEES BEND (Number 16, page 112)

A loaded barbell is placed across your shoulders, or taken by you from the stands made for this purpose. You stand short astride toes pointing to the front. Feet should not be more than 18—24 inches apart. From this position and KEEPING THE BACK FLAT all the time, the knees are bent fully, or to the thighs parallel with the ground if you are not too supple in the hips. When you have assumed the lower position you return to the upright. Here again great care must be taken that the back remains flat and that the seat does not in any way come up first. It is incorrect rising from the knees bend position that can cause backaches and minor injuries. It is advisable to raise the heels on a block of wood about 2 inches high for this exercise, especially if you find that you cannot keep your heels on the floor when doing this exercise. With a block, more emphasis is thrown on the front part of the thighs, one of the weak spots in the make-up of many athletes.

The Squat not only strengthens all the thigh muscles, but has a very marked effect on the whole of the respiratory system, strong heart and lungs being of great importance to any athlete. Because of this effect the exercise is a great chest and stamina builder.

All events, whether field or track, call for strong leg work, and many an athlete has been let down with pulled or strained thigh muscles or cramp, more often than not because the muscles are not strong enough to take the strain imposed on them. Even throwing events are dependent on some form of co-ordinated leg work, either with a run up, or movement within a circle, and in all these events the initial drive originates from the legs.

The number of repetitions and poundages used must be varied slightly, according to the needs of the individual and the event.

For runners, I recommend high repetitions which combine strength with stamina and suggest three sets of 15 repetitions with a basic poundage of about 50 lb. For jumpers I recommend the same. For Field Events, I recommend slightly lower repetitions, particularly for the heavy events like shot and hammer, and suggest a basic weight of about 70 lb. to be varied according to need and experience, working up to anything like 200 lb. without impairing speed.

A good variation to this exercise is to rise very quickly and jump in the air slightly, but of course in this form you cannot use a block under the heels. However, it is a good exercise for sprinters, jumpers and hurdlers wanting a quick 'snap' to their muscles.

Breathing is very important in this exercise. A deep breath is taken just prior to the knees bend and held until the upright position is reached again. On regaining the upright position, several quick deep breaths are taken before the next repetition. The heavier the poundage used the more breaths are taken before each repetition. Don't restrict your breathing to the nose. Open your mouth too and get all the air you can.

THE STRAIGHT ARM PULLOVER AT ARMS' LENGTH (Number 4, page 108)

This is a natural follow on to the Squat. The name is self-explanatory, but I will describe the exercise and its purpose. It can be done on the floor, but preferably on a bench, as the height of the discs on the floor removes a great deal of the initial benefit on the deltoid and latissimus dorsi muscles.

Lie on a bench with the arms above your head holding a lightly loaded bar or swingbell (centrally loaded dumbell rod). I prefer the use of a swingbell for this exercise, as it is easier to control and better balanced for the more inexperienced person. From this position lower the weight behind the head, keeping the arms locked all the time, until the arms are in a straight line with the body. By lying towards the end of the bench, the arms are free of the bench at the extremities. Immediately the arms reach this position, pull the weight straight back to the starting position, still keeping the arms straight and elbows locked. This exercise should be executed fairly fast, and a light weight used. Here again breathing is most important. A deep breath is taken as the bar is lowered to arms outstretched position, and exhaled as the bar returns to overhead. Here again it is essential that no part of the back leaves the bench. This exercise also stretches the whole of the rib box in a more marked way than the Bench Press. It strengthens and gives mobility to the whole of the rib box, and gives a full range of movement to the shoulder girdle so necessary for any throwing event and even in the arm action of running.

I suggest high repetitions in this exercise 12—15 with about 15 lb. to commence.

The exercise can be made slightly stronger by taking the weight right to the thighs and then to arms' length behind the head and so covering a full range of movement 180 degrees with the weight.

THE BENCH PRESS (Number 6, page 109)

You lie on a bench or form not more than 18 inches to 2 feet wide (so that the shoulders can move freely), and not higher than 2 ft. 6 in. It may have to be lower so that the feet are firmly placed on the floor on either side of the bench. The exercise can be done with the feet also on the bench, but the balance is poorer in this position. Take a bar to arms' length, or have it handed to you, and with a grip about 24—30 inches wide, according to the length of your arms, lower the weight to the chest, and then press it to arms' length and repeat. Breathe in deeply just as you begin to lower the bar to the chest and breathe out as the bar reaches the arms' length position again.

An essential point to remember is that the back remains flat on the bench throughout the movement. The merits of this exercise are that it is a great chest and stamina builder, and that it can be performed with heavy weights without any fear of injury or muscle trouble. It exercises the whole of the thoracic cavity and so has a very marked effect on the respiratory system. For stamina building in particular, I recommend high repetitions with a light weight.

Besides exercising the respiratory system, it exercises the pectorals, triceps, deltoids, and trapezius. All these muscles are used in the throwing events, and particularly in the pole vault.

I suggest that for field events a rather higher poundage is used with lower repetitions. For runners I suggest that three sets of 12 repetitions commencing with about 50 lb. would make an average start, and for the field events and those who need some upper body development I suggest three sets of eight repetitions commencing with 70 lb. as an average.

These two exercises alone would form an excellent basis for all athletic and sporting events, whether during the athletic season or in the off season, and that they would combine excellently with any other form of training.

I consider however, that two more exercises would make a better basic schedule for all events, and cover every muscular requirement of the athlete. The other two as mentioned earlier, are:

THE GOOD MORNING EXERCISE (Number 9, page 110)

This is a simple exercise. You stand feet astride with a barbell supported across the shoulders. From this position bend the trunk forward until it is at right angles to the body and return to upright position.

Keep the head well back when bending to prevent the bar from slipping over the neck. If you are a bit tight in the hamstrings, try to go lower than right angles, but be careful not to overbalance.

This is an excellent lower back exercise, and also a good one for the back of the thighs so essential to runners and jumpers.

The lower back is a very vulnerable spot, and, if weak, the seat of many minor aches and pains. It is the pivoting point and centre of gravity for all field events.

I suggest three sets of 10 repetitions for this exercise, commencing with a poundage of about 30 lb.

As a substitute for the Good Morning Exercise, the DEAD LIFT is also a good exercise, especially for the events demanding strength.

The DEAD LIFT is done by standing close to a fairly heavily loaded barbell, and by bending the knees and keeping the back perfectly flat and arms straight, lift the weight off the floor until you are standing upright. For comfort one hand is placed overgrasp on the bar, and one undergrasp. This is an excellent back and leg strengthener, and can be done with legs straight as a very advanced lower back exercise. I suggest low repetitions about three sets of 6, with about 140 lb. for this exercise.

Every athlete should devote ample time to development of strength in the abdominal region.

Supple and strong abdominal muscles are essential for all events, and generally speaking freestanding abdominal work will be sufficient to keep the muscles well toned. Such exercises as Back Lying Arms Above the Head, legs raise, and Sit-Ups are old favourites. Also the Back Lying Hips Support alternate leg swings, and the cycling action. In addition there should be plenty of trunk side bending, twisting, lunging, high kicks, and all round suppling exercises.

Some work with Iron Boots will be invaluable for all events. All the freestanding abdominal exercises can be done with iron boots for added resistance. Fitted with a dumbell certain excellent leg exercises can be done, particularly for weak knee joints and thigh muscles. Back curls done in standing position with Iron Boots fitted with dumbells are ideal for the sprinter and jumper, and the seated thigh extension is excellent for the quadriceps and strengthening the knee joint. It is a popular exercise with footballers recovering from cartilage operations.

Where there is weakness in the actual muscles used for a particular event, I recommend these exercises:

SPRINTING

Some extra Iron Boot work for the calf muscles, such as Back Curls and Calf Raises. Some leg extensions with Iron Boot and dumbell attachments.

To improve the arm action, ALTERNATE DUMBELL PRESS—Stand astride with a light dumbell held at each shoulder, press them alternately overhead with plenty of snap in the final position. As one dumbell begins to lower, commence pressing the other one. I suggest three sets of 8 repetitions each side, with a weight around 15 lb. each dumbell for a start.

MIDDLE DISTANCE RUNNERS

The Dumbell Press as above. Also some extra abdominal work with iron boots. Here is a good extra abdominal exercise. Sit with hands support behind you, knees raise high to chest and lower. Try three sets of 12 repetitions with Iron Boots.

Cramp is often the bogey of middle and long distance runners and this one exercise alone should help prevent it occurring.

POLE VAULT

A good pole vaulter has to be quite a good acrobat to complete the evolutions necessary in mid-air for anything like a good championship height. He must be agile and very strong in the arms, shoulders, abdominals and trunk. He needs added strength in the arms to pull himself up on the pendulum swing, and his heaving muscles must be particularly strong. I recommend the following exercises for the pole vaulter:

Curls. Stand feet short astride holding a barbell at arms' length, with the hands in the undergrasp position. The distance between the hands should not be more than shoulder width. Without any body motion, curl the bar upwards, by contracting and using the upper arm muscles. Lift the shoulders slightly to complete the movement. I suggest three sets of 10 repetitions with around 60 lb. to begin with.

Sidebends with Dumbells. Stand astride grasping a dumbell in each hand. Trunk bend from side to side lifting the dumbell up and under on the opposite side to the bend. I suggest three sets to a count of 16 with 10 lb. on each dumbell to commence.

Chinning. Hanging overgrasp on a bar or beam, fairly wide grip with the hands, do as many pull ups as possible. Three sets of 8—10 repetitions. Ensure that the feet do not come forward.

If facilities permit, pulley work would also be useful for this event.

JAVELIN

Great speed and co-ordination are needed for this event, and a strong and very supple shoulder girdle. Extra deltoid and triceps work would be an asset, besides of course the basic exercises.

The Pullover at Arms' length, one of the Basic Exercises already described, is excellent for this event, but instead of taking the weight only to arms' length, carry the weight right down to the thighs and back, describing a complete half circle with the arms. This ensures a full range of movement for the shoulder girdle.

The Alternate Dumbell Press already described for Sprinting, is also a good deltoid strengthener.

One last exercise: THE SINGLE ARM SWING WITH DUMBELL —Take a light dumbell. Stand feet astride knees bent with the dumbell held at arms' length between the feet. Swing the dumbell to overhead, straightening the knees at the same time. Repeat

145

both sides. I suggest three sets of 10 repetitions with 10 lb. dumbell as a start.

DISCUS

Speed and co-ordination are also necessary here, within the confines of a small circle. Great drive is needed, commencing from the legs.

The basic exercises are almost sufficient to cover this, but I suggest the Dumbell Swing, as for Javelin, as a good extra exercise.

Strong Oblique muscles are also very necessary; for this I suggest the Sidebends with Dumbells, as recommended for the Pole Vault, and also this one: TRUNK TWIST WITH BARBELL—Stand astride with a barbell across the shoulders—twist the body from left to right as far as possible, trying to keep the hips square to the front. I suggest three sets of 10 repetitions each way with a trial weight of 30 lb.

PUTTING THE SHOT

Although speed and co-ordination are essential, the heavier athlete is usually best suited to this event, with height a great advantage. The basic exercises should cover most requirements, but I also suggest the Swing with dumbells as for Javelin and Discus, and the Alternate Dumbell Press as described for Sprinting.

The final thrust with the fingers in this event is very important, and to strengthen the fingers the ordinary Dips or Press-ups on the floor but done on the finger tips, instead of the flat of hand, will be very helpful. Heavier weights can also be used in the Squat.

THE HAMMER

This is definitely a strong man's event, and great speed is needed. The basic exercises should cover the requirements, but use added weight and also the Dead Lift, already described, instead of the Good Morning Exercise. For added shoulder strength, add the Alternate Dumbell Press, already described for Sprinting.

One other suggested exercise is UPRIGHT ROWING—Hold a bar at arm hang position, feet astride, narrow grip. Without leaning the body, lift the bar as high up the front of the body as possible, bending the elbows outwards, and lower. I suggest three sets of 10 repetitions, commencing with 30 lb. as a trial.

HOP, STEP AND JUMP

The triple jump calls for speed and co-ordination, great back and abdominal strength. The basic exercises should cover all the requirements, but I suggest that the Dead Lift is used instead of the Good Morning Exercise, both described in the Basic Exercises. Additional abdominal work should be undertaken, preferably with Iron Boots. I suggest Sitting Hands Support—Knees raise high to chest. Three sets of as many repetitions as possible. Also back lying hips support, alternate leg swing with, Iron Boots.

HIGH JUMP

The modern styles of High Jump, like the pole vault, call not only for strong and resilient muscles, but a certain amount of acrobatic ability and lots of suppleness in the hip. The basic exercises should be sufficient for strength, but we also suggest Iron Boot work for abdominals as for the triple jump, and in addition; High kicks with Iron Boots, Back leg swings with Iron Boots, Back lying legs raise a foot off the floor, legs swing apart and close. I suggest three sets of 15 repetitions if possible for this. These should cover requirements for the Straddle or the Eastern Cut Off and Western Roll methods.

Weights Give the Sportsman that Extra Lift

LONG JUMP

Speed and leg strength and strong abdominals are needed for this event, whether for the Hitch Kick style or the Sail Flight. The basic exercises should be sufficient, with Jumping Squats already described. Iron Boot work and abdominal work described for Hop, Step and Jump will also be beneficial.

Remember that sprint training is as important as the actual jump.

Many of the exercises suggested for the various athletic events are also suitable for all other sports, and for the sports specialist who needs some extra work to promote added strength and stamina.

I must assure my readers that weight training exercises definitely help other sports, particularly in the off season. Correctly applied, they will keep the sportsman fit all the year round. I can name countless top line sportsmen who have used and benefited from progressive resistance exercises, though it may not be generally known that they have used this type of training. Top line footballers, golfers, swimmers, divers, and tennis players, in fact sportsmen of every kind, have taken to weight training for improving their power for their own sport. One or two complete football clubs have tried out weight training quite successfully.

It is quite obvious that stronger muscles would greatly eliminate the number of injuries sportsmen sustain, footballers in particular, where certainly the chances of knee and joint injuries would be greatly lessened.

Most sports have a one-sided effect on the body resulting in lack of balance, and certain muscles are developed at the expense of others, particularly in the specialist. The majority of sports give play to the legs more than to any other part of the body. Games with bat or racquet or club develop a lop-sided physique and must be balanced up by a properly planned exercise schedule.

148

Weights Give the Sportsman that Extra Lift

Abdominal work is of primary importance in all sports, and should really be automatically included in the basic exercises. Weak abdominals reduce stamina and promote fatigue, back aches, etc., and leave you prone to many minor injuries.

Such exercises as Back lying, arms above the head, legs raise; Back lying, sit ups; Back lying, hips support alternate leg swings to touch floor behind head; Back lying legs raise 6 inches and from this position, legs part and close, should be included in all workouts for sport, along with limbering up, skipping, running etc. Side bends, trunk twisting, toe touching, etc., should also be included.

If these exercises become monotonous, do them with Iron Boots. You get greater resistance in less time this way.

A footballer needs particularly strong abdominals for heading, twisting and turning at speed. A boxer needs them to withstand the body blows he receives and to stand up to the terrific demands on stamina. In fact, no athlete should neglect his abdominals. They must be as hard as steel in contraction and as supple as rubber when relaxed.

The four basic exercises recommended for athletics are ideally suited for all sports, but I must add one more, which I think is an ideal upper body and back strengthener.

This exercise also counteracts the possibility of postural defects in games which entail rather a lot of crouching, or one-sided work. It also helps to develop the triceps muscles and wrists so essential to the bat and racquet games. The exercise is:

The Press Behind Neck

Stand astride, with a barbell across your shoulders behind the neck. From this starting position, press the bar overhead, without any jerk or body movement. All the upper back muscles come into play, and the triceps of the upper arm. This being a very strong exercise, I suggest for the beginner three sets of 8 repetitions with 40 lb. as a trial weight. Take a deep breath prior to the press and exhale as you lower the weight. Ensure that the bar touches the top of the spine at the end of each movement.

FOOTBALL

Two special exercises might well be used by all footballers.

A good arm exercise would be beneficial, since there is little play on these during a game. I suggest the CURL WITH BARBELL. Stand astride, hold a bar at the hang position, fairly narrow grip. Without any body movement, and by contracting the upper arm muscles, curl the bar upwards until the knuckles touch the shoulders, lifting the elbows well up. I suggest three sets of 8 repetitions with 50 lb. for a trial.

If there is a weakness in the quadriceps of the thigh, do some extra Iron Boot work with dumbell fittings. Include THIGH EXTENSION. Sit on a high table or bench, and alternate leg stretch forward. This is also a wonderful exercise for strengthening the whole of the knee joint.

Some extra calf work may also be necessary for footballers, and this might take the form of seated with barbell across knee, and toes on a block of wood, heels raise from this position. Ordinary freestanding calf raises with toes on a block will also be beneficial.

With barbell across knees I suggest 3 sets of 15 repetitions with 120 lb. as a trial.

RUGBY

There is less actual footwork in rugby, but the needs will be the same. Wing three-quarters would do well to use the exercises prescribed in the training for sprinters. Forwards need plenty of arm and shoulder strength as well as powerful legs for pushing in the scrum. I would recommend rather heavier squats for them, and the basic exercises. Some added chinning or work on a pulley, particularly Kneeling Pull Behind Neck would be beneficial.

CRICKET

There may seem no connection whatever between cricket and weight training, but I feel sure that some added strength would greatly help the cricketer and relieve fatigue when fielding or batting for long hours. Strong abdominals are essential, as are strong legs, shoulders and arms.

I consider the basic exercises carried out, with Dead Lift added, should serve admirably to get and keep a cricketer fit in the off season.

BOXING

Most boxers, except the Heavyweights, have to try and keep their weight down, so any weight training for those with weight troubles would need to be on the light side with plenty of repetitions. The basic exercises are quite suitable, with extra emphasis on abdominal work. The squats would have to be done quickly with light weights.

. In addition, I suggest some extra arm and shoulder work for more power. Add the Alternate Dumbell Press already explained as for sprinting, also with very light dumbells 5 to 10 lb. each, try going through the punching action.

THE REVERSE CURL should also be added for greater forearm strength. This is done exactly the same as the curl, described for Football, but with the knuckles uppermost, and the weight only taken to right angles with the body. This is a tougher exercise than the curl and I suggest three sets of 10 repetitions with 30 lb. for a trial.

A boxer is often let down by his legs, and extra emphasis on leg work would work wonders. For the squats try sets of 20 repetitions instead of the 10 to 12 usually quoted.

If good style and technique can be obtained fast Snatching a weight from floor to arms' length overhead would prove an effective all round exercise.

CYCLING

More and more racing cyclists have in the past two years trained with weights, particularly in the off season. Both sprinters and long distance cyclists have benefited greatly through weight training, and the official cycling journals have often advocated weight training exercises.

Apart from leg work, many cyclists are in great need of some upper body work, particularly for the chest and rib box.

The basic exercises are ideally suited for this, particularly the Straight Arm Pullover and the Bench Press. The Press Behind Neck will counteract the bad effect of continued stooping over handle bars, and the Good Morning Exercise and Dead Lift, will be invaluable for lower back strength so essential in a gruelling race.

Most cyclists have more than enough leg work, but the squat will add power and strength to their legs. They should also do the Iron Boot exercises recommended for Footballers.

If facilities permit, and there is a suitable leg pressing machine, this will also be ideal for the cyclist. I suggest four sets of 10 repetitions starting with about 170 lb. as a trial where leg pressing facilities exist.

I know of a champion cyclist who trained only on three exercises: Squats, Bench Press and Dead Lifts, with wonderful effect.

FENCING

Most good fencers usually have superbly developed thighs, and therefore do not need much extra work, but some additional squatting would not be out of place and particularly some calf work, as the movements of fencing do not bring the calf muscles greatly into play. Freestanding calf raises, as recommended for football, are indicated, also the bar across knees seated calf raise already described is a useful exercise.

Weights Give the Sportsman that Extra Lift

If leg strength should be weak try lunges with a barbell held across shoulders. Stand feet together, with a barbell across shoulders, lunge forward first with the right foot, then with the left, alternately, going into a deep lunge as for fencing, hold the position for a few seconds before recovering. Try three sets of 8 repetitions each leg with a trial weight of 30 lb. across the shoulders.

Supple wrists and strong forearms are also needed, and some upper body and chest work. The basic exercises will fulfil this, and the Reverse Curl as described for Boxing. The barbell curl will be an added help, described in football training.

TENNIS AND SQUASH

Both these sports need great speed and tough resilient muscles, with split-second timing. There is less overhead work in Squash, but the essentials are similar. The basic exercises should supply the needs, with perhaps one or two extra arm and shoulder exercises to counteract the rather one-sided effect of holding a racquet.

I suggest that the ALTERNATE DUMBELL PRESS as described in sprinting should be added, also the REVERSE CURL described for boxing.

SIDEBENDS WITH DUMBELLS already described would help to promote strength to withstand the twisting and turning of Tennis and Squash.

BADMINTON

This sport calls for more overhead work than tennis and squash, and is played with a lighter racquet needing more delicate wrist work.

The basic exercises should be quite sufficient with perhaps the ALTERNATE DUMBELL PRESS added and the CURL as an extra arm exercise.

153

SWIMMING

Swimmers usually have long supple muscles, but some extra resistance work for strength and stamina would be beneficial. A powerful pull with the arms is needed for crawl, breast or the modern butterfly stroke. If facilities permit some extra pulley work would be very helpful for the swimmer. I suggest the DOWNWARD PULL TO BACK OF NECK in kneeling position. This is a great exercise for the latissimus dorsi group, used for pulling. As an alternative some overgrasp CHINNING or Pull Ups on a bar or beam would be helpful. Use fairly wide grip, and ensure that the feet and legs are kept well back.

For the legs, nothing could be better than practising your leg stroke whether for breast stroke or crawl, wearing Iron Boots, and lying across a form supporting yourself on your hands. Back lying alternate legs swing with hips support and wearing Iron Boots would also help, and back lying legs raise slightly and legs parting.

ROWING

The basic exercises should cover the requirements, but extra arm and shoulder work, strong abdominals, and thighs, with a tough lower back are all essentials to the oarsman. I would add UPRIGHT ROWING—it has already been described in the athletics training for the Hammer. I suggest again three sets of 10 repetitions with 30 lb.

The CURL WITH BARBELL should also be added and plenty of iron boot work for really tough abdominals.

If facilities exist, the LEG PRESS would also be a useful addition, if not some STRADDLE LIFTS—this is done by standing astride a bar, with one hand held in front of the body and one in the rear. Ensure that the bar is balanced. Bend the knees and pick the bar up, and keeping the back flat, bend and stretch the knees in this position, keeping arms straight. I suggest three sets of 10 repetitions with about 120 lb. as a trial.

HOCKEY

The basic exercises should cover the requirements for this fast sport, with some extra arm and shoulder work if a player finds these tire quickly.

BASKET BALL

This game has become very popular in recent years even in this country and is one of the fastest and most strenuous games when played by crack teams. Heaps of stamina and split-second timing are needed. Most of its best players are tall and slim, so some upper body work is always indicated.

THE ALTERNATE DUMBELL PRESS already described, should be added, while for some extra arm work (since the arms do not get a great deal of actual strengthening work) the CURL WITH BARBELL should be added. The Jumping Squat would be better than the ordinary squat for players of this particular sport.

NOTE: *In the following chapter on Breathing some exercises are given which every bodybuilder can do with advantage to health and physique. But the author wants to make it clear that modern breathing exercises for particular respiratory troubles and chest conditions are nearly always of the localized type: Diaphragmatic, Costal and Apical, taken from suitable starting positions, e.g. Crook Lying (Figure 11, page 58). In these cases arm movements are seldom employed, because the muscles responsible for raising the arms restrict (by fixator action) the movements of the ribs.*

CHAPTER FOURTEEN

Take a Second Look at Your Breathing

It is not generally appreciated that breathing is the most important function and action of the human body. We can do without food, water, sleep, exercise for several days but stop the action of breathing for a spell and life goes.

It is unfortunately true that because of the sheltered and sedentary lives people live nowadays very few indeed breathe correctly and so go through life in a sort of air-starved condition which shows itself in pale faces, hollow eyes, poor complexions and general lassitude, conditions which disappear miraculously when sensible outdoor exercise is taken up.

To the bodybuilder correct breathing is all important. As he performs his exercises, an increased flow of blood is directed to his muscles. Waste products which are formed must be pumped by the heart to the lungs for reconditioning and filtration. His lungs must necessarily work much harder and because it is vitally important that he should never reach the stage of complete breathlessness, which may result in giddiness or blackouts, the bodybuilder will find that in many exercises breathing through the nose is insufficient. He will find that if he does the exercises correctly, he must not only take great gulps of air through his mouth, but that breathing must become as important as the actual exercise.

It is very necessary then, during a training session in which a good deal of mouth breathing takes place, that the air in the gym or training quarters should be as clean and fresh as possible. The nasal organs work almost perfectly as filters of dust and germs but the mouth and throat have no such protection. Training in a polluted atmosphere can result therefore in trouble in the respiratory system, unless care is taken.

It is always advisable to end a training session with a few breathing exercises which help to bring about a slowing down of the flow of blood. Specialists call this the 'tapering off' and it is just as important as the original 'warming up'.

Here are a few exercises which will give much help to achieve better mobility of the chest.

1. Stand astride (preferably in an atmosphere of fresh but not cold air), arms circling slowly forward and upward to brush past ears and slowly down. Make a complete circle with the arms. Breathe in slowly through the nose on the upward movements and out on the downward. Fingers stretched. Repeat slowly 12 to 15 times.

2. Stand astride, arms raise sideways and upwards to overhead till fingers touch, lower slowly. Breathe in slowly on upward movement, out on lower, inhaling through nose and exhaling through mouth or nose. Repeat 12 times.

3. Back lying, arms sideways, palms of hands flat on floor, knees up, feet on floor. Chest lift off floor, breathe in slowly on lift, breathe out on lower. Repeat 12 times.

4. Stand astride, hands on lower ribs well spread out. Breathe in slowly through the nose, feeling 'flaring of ribs', and slight abdominal distension at beginning, and lift head slightly back. Breathe out slowly. Repeat 12 times.

5. Stand astride, arms forward, fingers pointed. Arms part slowly breathing in, force shoulder blades well back. Return to starting position breathing out.

6. Back lying, knees raise, feet flat on floor, palms of hands on floor at sides—Breathe in and out, slowly drawing in abdomen and lifting chest, breathe out slowly.

CHAPTER FIFTEEN

Coming to Terms with Weight Training

There are many terms and abbreviations used in modern bodybuilding which may confuse a beginner. I have already explained some of the training terms in this book, but for easy reference I list briefly some of those which have already been mentioned, and which you will often see repeated many times in physical culture journals.

To the layman, many of the terms may be quite strange and meaningless. Most of the modern bodybuilding terms originated in the U.S.A. and were coined for easy reference. I have tried in this book not to use abbreviations, which I consider slipshod, particularly when referring to muscles, but as you are likely to come across them very often in physical culture journals and in clubs, I will mention a few:

Muscle Abbreviations
'TRAPS.' The Trapezius Muscles.
'PECS.' The Pectoralis Muscles.
'DELTS.' The Deltoids.
'CEPS.' The Biceps of Upper Arm.
'LATS.' The Latissimus Dorsi Muscles.

General Terms
BODYBUILDING. The science of improving your physique by all

forms of exercise but particularly with progressive resistance exercises.

BULK. The term used to describe added muscle weight, which is required, rather than fat, of which people want to rid themselves.

DEFINITION OR 'CUTS'. The term given to quality of muscle formation rather than quantity. People who have thin skins, without any fatty tissue over the muscles, are said to have good 'Definition'. Care with diet, decrease of liquids, and higher repetitions help to improve definition.

MUSCLE BOUND. A very misused term for those who train with resistance exercise, but seldom found in those who follow correct training methods. Through over use of 'cramped' muscles, a person can become 'tight' or muscle bound. In this way the uneven pull of muscles restricts full movement of joints. Certain occupations are far more likely to produce this condition than progressive exercise.

MUSCLE CONTROL. This is the static contraction and relaxation of muscle groups by will power, and the isolation of certain muscle groups. It requires great concentration and practice, and is a fine way of keeping the muscles toned up.

REPETITIONS. Often abbreviated to 'REPS', is the number of consecutive times you do each exercise without a break. Usually 8—10.

REST PERIOD. The short rest or 'Breather' taken between each Set of exercises, or between each exercise.

SCHEDULE. The term given to a specified plan of training. The exercises you will do, the number of repetitions, etc.

SETS. When you have performed a specified number of repetitions, you have done one SET.

SET SYSTEM. This is the method generally recommended, whereby you do a specific number of SETS of each exercise before passing on to the next one. The most popular method generally is to do THREE SETS OF EACH EXERCISE 8—10

REPETITIONS. Abbreviated it is written like this 3 × 8 Reps. or 8 × 8 × 8.

SPECIALIZED SCHEDULES. Those schedules done for special remedial purposes or by advanced bodybuilders, who are specializing on specific parts of the body where there are flaws in their physique, or weakness in certain muscle groups.

WEIGHT LIFTING. A competitive sport recognized by the Olympic Games, whereby competitors in various classes of bodyweight, lift their maximum weight on certain recognized lifts.

WEIGHT TRAINING. The use of barbells, dumbells and weights for progressive exercise.

WORKOUT. A training session.

The terminology of many of the exercises are often abbreviated and difficult for a beginner to follow:

Abbreviation of Exercise Names

C. & J. Clean and Jerk (one of the Olympic Lifts).

D.K.B. The Deep Knee Bend of the Squat.

P.O.A.L. The Pullover at Arms' Length or Straight Arm Pullover.

P.O.B. Press on Back.

T.H. Two hands, often appears as a part of the description of an exercise.

These are about the main abbreviations you are likely to see, though of course all the exercises could be similarly abbreviated.

Terms Applied to Various Methods of Training

CHEATING. The method used by advanced bodybuilders to force up the weights used at the expense of style.

CRAMPING. Half range movements, which concentrate on contracting and enlarging the muscles, without working a full range. Cramping can also be done statically with some muscles by repetition contraction, like the Biceps, without fully relaxing them between movements.

DOUBLE PROGRESSION. Here you increase the number of sets *and* the number of repetitions during a specified period.

FLUSHING. All the exercises are concentrated to one area of the body and done consecutively, before going on to another part. In other words, all upper body, or arm exercises, are done before moving on to the lower half of the body. The exercises are also speeded, so that the blood supply is increased to certain areas.

MULTI-POUNDAGE SYSTEM. The bar is loaded with a given weight, and as many repetitions as possible are done with it, until fatigue makes it impossible to do more. Two discs are then removed, and the exercise continued without a break, until it is impossible to do any more repetitions, even though the original weight has been greatly lowered. Not a great many repetitions are possible even with this method.

ONE AND A HALF METHOD. A full range movement is done in a set of repetitions, followed by a half range movement. For instance, when doing a Curl, you do a full range curl from the starting position, and then instead of lowering the weight to the starting position for the next repetition, you lower it half way, only working the middle and outer range of movement every second repetition. This method can be employed with many exercises in advanced bodybuilding, and is a tough one.

PUMPING. Done usually prior to a physique contest, so that the muscles are temporarily enlarged, by quick, light repetitions of short range movements.

REBOUND METHOD. Another method of cheating on certain exercises to enable you to handle heavier weights. The weight is made to rebound off the floor, chest, or bench, when doing repetitions to give you an initial start. It can be used for Bench Press, Pullover or even Squats, when you go down very quickly, and bounce up.

Coming to Terms with Weight Training

SET PROGRESSION. Is when you increase the number of Sets of any exercise. You may decide to do three Sets, and over a period of weeks to increase to five sets, still doing the original number of repetitions.

SUPER SETS. You work two exercises alternately, doing one set of one, then one set of the other, until the required number of sets are completed. If working the arms for instance, you can use an exercise primarily for biceps, followed by one for the triceps. In this way you exercise certain muscle groups and their antagonistic groups immediately afterwards.

CHAPTER SIXTEEN

Weight Training for Boys

Are weight training exercises suitable for boys, and if so, at what age is it safe for them to start? These are two questions often put to the author. My answer is always this. There is no reason at all why young boys should not benefit from progressive weight training exercises, providing SUCH EXERCISES ARE CAREFULLY SUPERVISED BY A KNOWLEDGEABLE PARENT OR A COMPETENT INSTRUCTOR. Each boy must be treated as an individual according to his capabilities. There can be no generalizations.

There is no standard bodybuilding course for boys. That is why it is better NOT to encourage all boys to do this type of exercise, because so many join clubs which have no qualified instructor and are just allowed to go their own way with what may be disastrous results in later life.

Most boys nowadays get some form of Physical Education at school and nearly always adequate facilities for games. Many schools in big towns have organized swimming. It is best to encourage boys to follow these *normal adolescent activities*. I consider that any form of weight training for boys should be done more in the nature of remedial work to strengthen a fast-growing boy, or to improve posture or minor defects, rather than as an alternative to the normal activities a boy should be encouraged to follow. It is not always a good thing for a young boy to emulate his older brother's strength feats, which may lead to a too-early desire to see how big he can get.

163

Weight Training for Boys

Youthful enthusiasm needs careful watching. The young boy is often too anxious to look like the muscular photograph he sees in physical culture magazines and his imagination can run riot. Many a young lad tags on to an older lad, who himself has little idea what he is doing, and in no time the exercises are being done incorrectly, and with one object in mind, to grow bulging muscles. Minor postural defects are soon aggravated, and growing bones are pulled out of position. Another factor which needs watching is the sense of rivalry between boys. If they are left on their own it is only natural they will want to see how much weight they can handle, so that they can beat their friends.

If boys are to handle weights, the instructor should have a good knowledge of each boy's capabilities, and should lay down for him the exact poundage to be used for each exercise.

The late Professor Edmond Desbonnet, the famous French physical culture authority, devised a method widely used in France which would work ideally with boys. He called it Weight Training in Class Formation, with each pupil doing the same exercise under an instructor, *but using varying sized barbells with varying weight, according to the capabilities of the individual.* Such classes would be ideal for boys, who would then be under the vigilant eye of an instructor, who could introduce a competitive spirit as the exercises were being done. He could also correct faulty positions and ensure perfect execution of each exercise.

Experiments have been carried out by education authorities in Sweden with weight training exercises with boys as young as nine years of age with splendid results. But Sweden has a long tradition of teaching exercises and the whole experiment is very carefully conducted.

There has been a big advance in this country too, and schools and Youth Clubs now include weight training in their P.E. programmes.

Weight Training for Boys

It is very essential that all weight training exercises done by boys should be selected from those with a full range of movement, and that great stress is made of correct starting positions and breathing, and that each movement is completely executed. Because of this, weights handled must always be well within the boy's capabilities to complete the required number of repetitions without any loss of form, and without any undue strain or restriction of normal breathing.

I will not attempt to suggest any poundages to be used by boys of a given age, because that varies so much even with boys of the same age. But I must stress, that except in the case of an exceptionally strong boy, and there are, of course, many, weights used must be of VERY LOW poundage.

For boys of 9—14 many of the pulley exercises already described in an earlier chapter would be suitable, particularly the SEATED PULL TO CHEST, AND THE SEATED PULL BEHIND NECK. I suggest the seated form of these two, as correct posture is easier to control when the exercise is done this way. Single arm pulley work is also suitable and would be interesting to a boy. Dip or Press ups done on the floor are also suitable as a further resistance exercise, provided that no body sag is permitted.

Any form of weight training or resistance work for boys should be part of *a complete training plan*, in which many freestanding exercises are also included, particularly prior to the weight training. Freestanding abdominal exercises should also play an important part. Most of those already prescribed would be quite suitable, provided that the number of repetitions is not more than TEN without a break. I suggest that abdominal exercises should be taken from the following :

1. Back lying—alternate knee raise to chest. Arms at sides, palms of hands flat on floor.

2. Same starting position with arms at sides—head lift off floor and toes turning upwards to look at feet.

3. Back lying—alternate leg raise.

4. Back lying arms above head—both knees raise high to chest.

5. Back lying arms above head—with ankle support—trunk raise to forward reach to put head on knees, keeping knees straight.

6. Back lying arms to sides, palms of hands on floor—both legs raise 45 degrees and lower.

I suggest that the following exercises are suitable, and under the conditions I recommend in this chapter would be beneficial for posture and general improvement in strength and the respiratory system:

PRESS BEHIND NECK (Ex. 3).

SQUAT WITH WEIGHT HELD AT CHEST, HEELS ON A BLOCK OF WOOD (Ex. 17).

STRAIGHT ARM PULLOVER WITH SWINGBELL (Ex. 45).

BENCH PRESS (Ex. 6).

GOOD MORNING EXERCISE (Ex. 9).

CURL WITH SWINGBELL (Ex. 49).

UPRIGHT ROWING (Ex. 7).

I think that these seven exercises are quite sufficient as part of a table for any boy up to the age of 14. I have deliberately avoided any exercises which may tend to compress a growing spine, or those which may cause a growing boy to hollow or round his back. I suggest that with ALL beginners, ONE SET OF SIX REPETITIONS of these exercises is quite sufficient, and that the number of repetitions can be increased to EIGHT as the boy advances, plus of course a slight increase in the weights used.

Boys over 12 can be advanced to TWO SETS of each exercise, if they have handled weights for over a year. Some boys of 14 are near adults, whereas some are still children, so care must be taken to gauge their training accordingly.

Weight Training for Boys

There are, of course, boys of exceptional physique at 14, who, if they are handled carefully, can do something more advanced.

I recommend that all boys up to 14 should do all their exercises with a short barbell of not more than 4 ft. 6 in. This will ensure better balance and execution of the exercises. A Swing-bell, too, is easier for a boy to handle.

Weights, when not in use, should be locked up and strict instructions should be given that they are not playthings but appliances which, if used carefully, can give them a safe route to sound healthy manhood and a strong physique which will help them in work and play.

CHAPTER SEVENTEEN

Figure Training for Women

Great strides have been made with resistance exercises for women in the past few years, and women from all walks of life and all age-groups have tasted the benefits of carefully planned resistance exercises to great advantage.

Weight training for women is not to be sneered at as something rather peculiar, or only for the athlete who may fail to pass the sex tests. There are as many modern health studios for women to-day as there are for men. In fact all the top studios cater for men and women on varying days. Naturally the approach is rather different, but many of the basic exercises are the same.

Modern health studios also cater for ladies with more of the specialized pieces of equipment such as gym bicycles, vibrators, rollers and other devices to attract them.

I had the privilege of looking after one of Britain's greatest ever tennis players for four months in 1967—Mrs. Ann Jones— at a time when, through injuries, etc., she had thought of retiring. Four months of weight training three times a week and she not only reached the Wimbledon finals, but went on to become a very successful professional. I believe she had no injuries to worry her for the reason she was doing regular resistance exercises at a well known London health studio under my supervision.

Because of the great strides made in this form of training for the busy woman, I have written a special book for the ladies,

Figure Training for Women

Modern Health and Figure Culture (Faber & Faber), if you want to go more deeply into the subject than a brief chapter in this book.

Weight training has for some years been accepted as standard practice for women athletes of all types, but especially for those whose events call for strength and stamina and muscular co-ordination. The benefits gained by the strengthening of the internal organs as well as the superficial musculature are tremendously important to every woman, and many of the exercises detailed for men can be practised by the fairer sex without causing any great difference in muscular size. No woman need fear that progressive resistance exercise will turn her into an Amazon.

It must be realized however that there are fundamental differences in a woman's anatomy which must be taken into account when planning suitable exercise. She is narrower in the shoulders, wider in the hips and, because of faulty posture caused by wearing unsuitable footwear, she often has a forward-tilted pelvis and a sway-back of the shoulders. She is often very flexible in the hips—particularly laterally—but weak in the lower back.

In the early part of training with light weights she should avoid all exercises where she carries weight overhead while she is in a standing position. She should concentrate on the figure correction exercises first—and do most of them lying down—before she goes into the stretch, swing and develop exercises which will do so much to improve fitness and the figure. The appliances required are not expensive. A steel bar, 4 feet long, two short dumbell rods and 4 collars and disc weights of these sizes will be enough: $4 \times 1\frac{1}{4}$ lb. discs, $4 \times 2\frac{1}{2}$ lb., 4×5 lb. and 2×10 lb. This will give a total weight when loaded on the bar of about 70 lb.—and this will only be used occasionally. Most of the work can be done with two dumbells weighing only 5–7½ lb. each.

A good training plan to follow would be 15–20 minutes in the evening before retiring, three times a week. A good uplift brassiere should be worn but very tight shoulder straps should be avoided. Brief under garments and a track suit are the ideal training clothing. After training take a warm shower or a good rub down with a rough towel. Avoid weight training exercise during the monthly period—substitute deep breathing exercises lying on the back with the knees supported on a high cushion or low stool instead.

Three different types of exercise programme are now described. The first—a conditioning course—is for normally healthy women who want to get a really good state of health. The second is specially designed to give uplift of the bust, more shapely shoulders and a better covering of flesh for an underweight person. And finally there is a brief course to follow for the woman who is overweight through lack of exercise. The very much overweight woman needs much more expert advice than can be given in instructions of a general nature.

One final point. In all the exercises avoid jerky movements and tensed-up positions. Do them smoothly and with a sense of natural rhythm, and DON'T USE WEIGHTS WHICH ARE TOO HEAVY to do the set number of exercises correctly.

Schedule 1: Ladies—Conditioning Course with Weights

Always loosen up with three to four minutes freestanding exercises before commencing your weight training. This will ensure complete mobility of the joints and avoid any muscular strains.

If you are a complete beginner and have not done any type of training previously, the Freestanding Exercises on pages 58 and 60 are perfectly suitable for ladies, i.e. The Toning Up Exercises for Beginners and the Intermediate ONLY, but OMIT Exercises 5 on page 58, and 6 on page 60 in these two schedules, and cut the repetitions down to about 10–12 in most exercises. Do these for about a fortnight before commencing your weight training. Later on use two or three of the exercises only as a general toning up prior to your weight training exercises.

GENERAL ADVICE

Initially do only ONE SET OF 10 REPETITIONS OF EACH EXERCISE but after three or four weeks when you find you are stronger progress to 2 SETS OF 8 REPETITIONS EACH EXERCISE. That is, you do *one* set, have a little breather, and repeat. All the exercises should be done correctly with special attention to correct breathing described in this book. No cheating or strain is necessary and though the weight used must be light, some real effort is needed.

DIET

Careful attention to diet is as essential for building up as it is for reducing. Read the chapter on diet, as the same things are applicable to you. Remember that the morning coffee habit can be ruinous to your figure. So is the 'little chat' over a cup of tea! Try to keep these to a pleasant minimum.

A good firm healthy figure built up by exercise is better than the best foundation garments.

1. Upright Rowing—Ex. 7, page 109. Illustration 7 on page 107. This is a fine chest, shoulder and upper body exercise. Maintain perfect posture throughout and see that the position of the body remains upright, with chin well up. Try 20 lb. as a start.

2. Straight Arm Pullover—done with a Swingbell—Ex. 4, page 108. Illustration Ex. 4, page 116. Women, being more supple than men in the shoulders, should ensure that the arms do not go too far beyond the straight line in the illustration or minor shoulder troubles may ensue: 7 lb. as a start. This is a great exercise for the rib box, respiratory system and also for uplift of the bust.

3. Bench Press—Ex. 6, page 109. Illustration Ex. 6, page 116. This is a fine all-round chest and shoulder exercise and one which enables even a girl to handle quite fair weights: 30 lb. as a start.

4. Good Morning Exercise—Ex. 9, page 110. Illustration 9, page 107. This is a fine lower back exercise, and because it counteracts the bad effect on the pelvis caused by wearing high heels, is a great posture and hip improver: 20 lb. as a start.

5. Squat—Ex. 16, page 112. Illustration Ex. 16, page 107. Before doing this exercise women should note several points. Always do the exercises with heels on a board or books about 2 in. high. Keep the knees well forward and not out sideways. The toes should point to the front and feet must not be too far apart. Ensure that the back is kept upright and controlled all the time. Do not squat too deeply and do not let the lower back sag. Try 30 lb. as a start.

6. Sidebend with Dumbell—Ex. 41, page 123. Illustration 41, page 107. This exercise should be done to a count of 20, that is bending ten times each way. It is a fine exercise for trimming the waist. Use a 10-lb. dumbell as a start.

Never neglect the abdominal exercises, do them first rather than miss them, as they are most important for good health. They should be taken from the Freestanding schedules on pages 58 and 60, Ex. 7 and 9. Also Ex. 9 on page 57. Illustration, page 58, Ex. 9. Try and do at least two and preferably three exercises for the mid-section each exercise session.

Schedule 2: Particularly for Uplift of Bust and Shoulder Improvement and Weight Gaining

Loosen up with some freestanding exercises, as before.

1. Alternate Dumbell Press—Ex. 23, page 117. Illustration, page 107, Ex. 23. This is a great shoulder exercise and should be done rhythmically. As one dumbell comes down the other goes up. No more than 5 lb. each dumbell for a trial. Repetitions as before.

2. Straight Arm Pullover. As in previous schedule, but this time take the weights right to the thighs and back to arms' length behind head. This not only improves the bust line but strengthens the shoulder girdle.

3. Bench Press—as before. Increase weight from previous schedule.

4. Flying Exercise with Dumbells—Ex. 27, page 117. Illustration, page 116, Ex. 27. This is a great exercise for making the bust firm, rounding and shaping it. No more than 5 lb. each dumbell for a start.

5. Squat—as before but increase repetitions to 12.

6. Straight-Legged Dead Lift—Ex. 10, page 110. Illustration, page 107, Ex. 10. A fine back strengthener, also excellent for hips and buttocks. Try with 30 lb.

7. Sidebends as before. Abdominals as before.

Schedule 3: All-Round Schedule with Emphasis on Reduction

Loosen up as before but include Freestanding Exercises 2 and 9 on page 59, and Ex. 2 and 3 on page 60.

1. Alternate Dumbell Press. As before, but increase number of repetitions to 12 each arm.

2. Upright Rowing. As in first schedule—2 SETS OF 8 REPETITIONS.

3. Straight Arm Pullover. As in first schedule but done more rapidly and 15 REPETITIONS. Use a lighter weight if necessary.

4. One Hand Swing—Ex. 30, page 118. Illustration, page 107, Ex. 30: 5–10 lb.

5. Flying Exercise with Dumbells. As in Schedule 2: 2 SETS OF 8 REPETITIONS.

6. Squats. As before but really light and done more rapidly: 15 REPETITIONS.

7. Good Morning Exercise. As in Schedule 1: 15 REPETITIONS.

8. Ex. 3, page 65 of Freestanding Schedule. Illustration, page 60.

9. Abdominal Work. From Freestanding Schedule, as before. Include Ex. 7, page 57. Illustration, page 58

CHAPTER EIGHTEEN

Now Exercise Your Will Power

Now you know all about weight training and what it can do for you. And you know that if you apply yourself to the task you will reap ample rewards. So off you go to grab hold of the nearest bar just loaded with weights. But hold on there. Just pause a little. Conserve some of this enthusiasm for the night when you think it is a little too cold. Or when you don't really feel up to it. When the television film interests you. That is when you want some of the enthusiasm and a dash of what all the champions have got—will power. Here's a quote you want to learn by heart. And remember. Mostly when you feel a bit jaded. Herb Elliott, the unbeaten Australian over a mile, said it: 'Anyone can train when he feels like it. But you have to keep training when you don't feel like it. You have to keep going at it all the time. Even when you're tired. That's what makes a champion. And that's what proves you're a man.'

Fitness is an elusive quality that you can acquire only by regular work-outs. Even those with the best intentions usually have lapses of interest. At the beginning these lapses are patched up. But there comes a time when the lapse stretches and the patching won't work. Here the best remedy is prevention. Just remind yourself what you want to achieve. Think about what you want to do. Then the enthusiasm will spurt back. Always keep your objective firmly in view. Think about it persistently; and stick to it tenaciously. For you can do anything you believe you can. And if you believe you can get weight training to help you then you will. It's only the nagging doubts that edge in at the corners of the mind; and they only loom up when you waver mentally from what you set out to do. So keep your objective right to the front with positive thoughts about it, and you will do whatever you want to do, because that basic thought is behind all the thinking of the top sportsmen in whatever sport you care to name. They may not realize that point immediately, but when you think about it that's what made them achieve what they did achieve—the thought that they did what they did because they thought they could.

In this book are all the weight training exercises that I consider necessary for you to become superbly fit. And in here are all the exercises that you need to become a Mr. Universe. You will have to use a little initiative and work out the schedule that you want for your needs. And after all, isn't that the basic requirement you want from life—getting what you particularly want? Now I have told you all you need to know about getting fit it's up to you. You are the one who has got to do it. No one can help you. All that talk about short cuts and special equipment and the magic formula is just not on. No one ever got anything for nothing. You are now required to work it out for yourself. There are quite capable men about who can pass on invaluable tips. But the end result depends on what you put in to it. All the very best luck. I hope you get what you want.

Index

Abdominal or endomorph, 26
Abdominal board, 92
Abdominal bulge, 25
Abdominal exercises, 63–4
Age factor, 20–4
Antagonist muscles, 32
Aponeuroses, 30
Appliances, weight training, 97–9

Barbell exercises, 103
Beginners' weight-training schedule, 115
Benches, types of, 90–1
Bench exercises, 92
Biceps, muscle, 33
Body-type, 25–8
Boys, weight training for, 163–7
Brachialis, muscle, 33
Breathing exercises, 57, 61, 63, 157
Build, measures of, 45–53
Bulge, abdominal, 25
Bulk, 159
Business man, weight training, 100

Calf exercise machine, 93
Carbohydrates, 40
Cardiac muscle, 30
Chair exercises, 72
Chest expansion, 47
Chest measurements, 48
Chinning bar, 86, 87
Classification of physique, 25–8

Concentric action, 31
'Cramping', explanation of, 160–1

Desbonnet system for boys, 164
'Definition', 159
Deltoid muscle, 106, 110
Diet, for bodybuilders, 38–44
Double progression, 161

Eccentric action, 31
Ectomorph, or thoracic, 26–7
Endomorph, or abdominal, 26
Epimysium, 31
Exercise, general plan, 55
Expander exercises, 76

Fats, in diet, 40
Feet exercises, 66–7
Figure training, for women, 168–74
Fixator muscles, 32
'Flushing', explanation of, 129–30, 161
Freestanding exercises (General), 58, 60, 62
Freestanding exercises (Mid-section), 63
Fulcrum, in muscle work, 34

Grip, to strengthen, 72

Habits, 18
Head harness, 93, 94
Health, 17

Index

Hippocrates, theory of type, 25

Insertion, of muscles, 30
Intermediate or mesomorph, 27
Involuntary muscle, 30
Iron boots, 87, 89
Iron boot exercises, 90
Isometric action, 31

Latissimus, muscle, 32
Leg press machine, 93, 94
Leverage, of muscles, 34–6
Levers, kinds of, 35

Measurements, average, 45
Measurements chart, 53
Measurements, how to take, 49, 50
Mechanics of muscle, 34
Medicine ball exercise, 73
Mesomorph or intermediate, 27
Minerals, in diet, 42
Multi-poundage system, 161
'Muscle binding', 36, 159
Muscle, construction of, 31
  Action of, 32
  Origin and insertion of, 30
  Types of, 30, 31

Olympic Games, 160
Origin, of muscles, 30

Parallel bars, 86
Pectoralis, muscle, 32
Perimysium, 31
Posture, 64
Posture exercises, 64
Power arm, 34, 35

Prime movers, 32
Proteins, sources of, 39
Pulley exercises, 83, 84
'Pumping', 161

Range of movement, 33
Rebound method, 161
Reducing exercises, for women, 174
Repetitions, 101
Resistance arm, 34
Resistance exercises without apparatus, 67–8
Roman chair, 91, 93
Roughage, in diet, 42

Sarcolemma, 31
Schedule, meaning and use, 99–102, 159–60
Schedules:
  Freestanding, 56–68
  Weight training, 132–4
Set system, 100–1
Shapes, of muscles, 31
Sheldon, Dr. William H., 25
Skipping, value of, 73
Snatch, two hands, 132
Squat stands, 94, 95
Super sets, 162
Swingbell exercises, 105
Synergist muscles, 32

Temperament, 25–8
Tendons, 30
Thoracic or ectomorph, 26
Toning up exercises (i), 56
Toning up exercises (ii), 59
Toning up exercises (iii), 61
Trapezius, muscle, 32

Type-training, 128

Ventilation, 70
Vitamins, 41
Voluntary muscle, 30

Wall exercises, 83
Wallbar exercises, 81, 89
Water, use of, 42
Weight training exercises (various), 103
Weight training for sportsmen:
  Badminton, 153

Basket ball, 155
Boxing, 151
Cricket, 151
Cycling, 152
Fencing, 152–3
Football, 150
Hockey, 155
Rowing, 154
Rugby, 150
Swimming, 154
Tennis and squash, 153
Workout, 160
Wrist roller, 72